Madness, Mayhem, and Modern Medicine

How in God's Creation Did We Get Here, and What Do We Do Now?

Madness, Mayhem, and Modern Medicine
How in God's Creation Did We Get Here, and What Do We Do Now?
Dr. L. H. Nelson

Paperback ISBN: 978-1-0881-1580-0

Hardcover ISBN: 978-1-0881-1588-6

PUBLISHED BY NXI PRESS
A DIVISION OF NICO 11 PUBLSIHING
MILWAUKEE, WISCONSIN

PRINTED IN THE UNITED STATES OF AMERICA

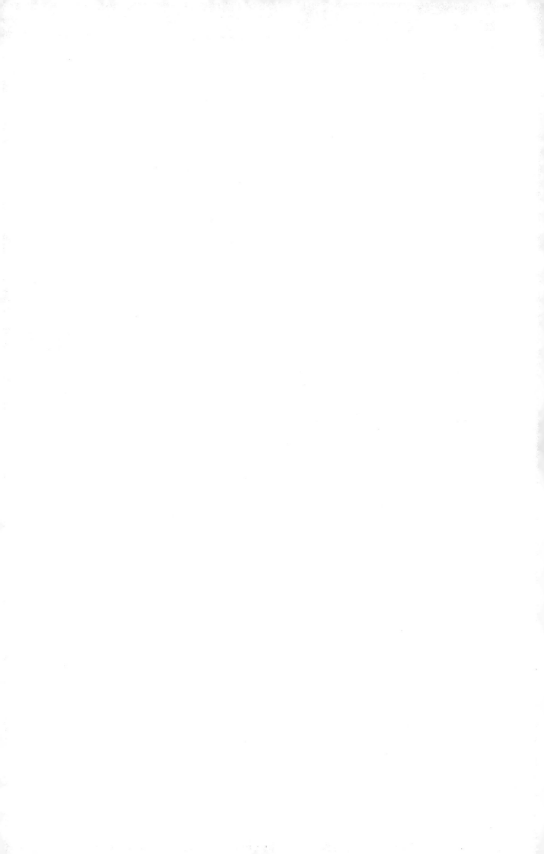

Dedicated to my mother and my father

TABLE OF CONTENTS

Part Two: What Happened

Part Three: What It Is Like Today

Now faith is the certainty of things hoped for,
a proof of things not seen.

Hebrews 11:1

Wonder With Me!

*Let's go to our Creator's Holy Throne together to glorify
Him in praise and thanksgiving!*

*Let's witness together the awesomeness of
His mysterious and spectacular creation!*

*And let's examine, as we stand shoulder to shoulder,
how we may have missed the mark in fending off the wiles of the enemy
as it seeks to devour and destroy what God had made for us.*

This is war!

Let's armor up together and get in the battle ...

~~~

*The Evil One, the Supreme Sorcerer, the Father of Lies,
continues to use magic and sorcery in a vain attempt to erase God's glory.
Is it using medicine as its weapon to annihilate mankind?*

~~~

*GOD is
the great "I AM"
the Alpha and the Omega, the Conqueror of all evil,
yesterday, today and forever.*

Preface

Is this world operating under the spell of the serpent? Is the practice of modern medicine filled with the sorcery of Satan? How deep does the deception go? How did we get here?

The evil devil dragon beckoned Eve to take one bite from the fruit of the forbidden tree, promising her that her eyes would be opened, she would be like God, all-knowing of good and of evil. How did the satanic serpent beguile and trick humanity over the ages?

Is the same ophidian tempting pharmaceutical minions and their servant physicians to bite from the same proverbial forbidden fruit, promising them profit, power, and a god-like status on earth? Is the media complicit? How deep does this debauchery go?

Eve said "yes" to the serpent.

It appears as though many have been tricked into saying "yes" to the same serpent, too. Doses of deadly medicines are doled out, transforming humans into slaves of pills at best, trans-humans at worst. Is the enemy swaying the newsmakers into spewing lies, and using preachers in the pulpits to convincingly utter its treacheries?

Have scientists and physicians unwittingly, or perhaps wittingly, become modern peddlers of medicinal magic? Do they even know? Just how soul sick have we become, really? Is there any hope for us?

Where are the clergy persons to tell us the truth about all of this? It seems as though this evil has spread and settled into the four corners of the earth.

Are we being poisoned by witchcraft? Just how deep is the devil's destruction of mankind? How broad is this trickery and deception?

Let's look and see, studying together exactly what has happened, and hear what God has to say about all of this ...

Strong's Concordance:

5331. Pharmakeia

pharmakeia: the use of medicine, drugs or spells
Original Word: φαρμακεία, ας, ἡ
Part of Speech: Noun, Feminine
Transliteration: pharmakeia
Phonetic Spelling: (far-mak-i'-ah)
Definition: the use of medicine, drugs or spells
Usage: magic, sorcery, enchantment.

pharmakeía (from pharmakeuō, "administer drugs") – properly,
drug-related sorcery, like the practice of magical-arts, etc.
(A. T. Robertson).

(https://biblehub.com/greek/5331.htm)

~~~

There shall not be found among you anyone
who makes his son or his daughter pass through the fire,
one who uses divination, a soothsayer, one who interprets omens,
or a sorcerer, or one who casts a spell, or a medium, or a spiritist,
or one who consults the dead.

For whoever does these things is detestable to the LORD;
and because of these detestable things
the LORD your God is going to drive them out before you.

Deuteronomy 18:10-12

Prologue

*Are you so foolish? Having begun by the Spirit,
are you now being perfected by the flesh?*

Galatians 3:3

December 2020

A masterful logician, a mind-bending magician, the enemy prowls among us, seeking to devour us all. Its hunger is never satiated. It's never satisfied. Heartless, it seeks, it destroys, it feeds its ego with the souls of distracted fools.

It took this long. A few thousand years. One second in eternity, a million moments on earth.

The enemy's lackeys were dispatched to confuse, mercilessly devouring the children first. The innocents, the defenseless, the babies. Then, it moved into the old, the feeble ones' homes, too. We didn't know their names, so we barely noticed they were gone. The babies had not even been named yet. Nameless, faceless, hidden in plain sight.

Mind games, sleight of hand, the enemy's magic show captivated us just enough to hypnotize our thoughts, enchant us, and capture our souls. Bewitched, we kept going back for more, not even realizing we had become its slaves.

We didn't notice the missing people until the dragon's tail had swept all of the defenseless into the mouth of the monster.

Somehow, we were so charmed that we didn't see past the tapping on the table. Entertained, we sat stupefied while we waited for the rabbit to hop out of the hat, never noticing the sinister plot in the kerchiefs, our thoughts drowned out in our thunderous applause when the rabbit finally appeared.

~ ~ ~

We started to notice something was amiss when our old aunties died. We recalled how they had hung their bedsheets outside on corded lines to dry in the sunshine. Their dainties were pinned on the lines hidden between the cotton sheets; their husband's white shirts fluttered in the breeze on the periphery. Everything picked up the glorious scent of the summer sun mixed with the fragrance of the flowers bending in the breeze nearby.

Time passed. Our aunties grew older and feeble, their frail fingers stashed the weathered wooden clothes pins in a corner junk drawer in the kitchen. They opted to toss their dainties and their bedsheets in the Maytag drying machines hidden in the dark corners of their basements.

These fragile, ancient aunties knew things, important things. We didn't even know the questions to ask them. Oh, they prattled on about this and that, while we listened with half of a lazy ear, more interested in pointing our feet in the direction of our next very important adventure.

Then, one day, they were gone.

It was then that we knew we should have paid more attention to what they had to say. Suddenly, we had so many questions, but realized their bag of answers tragically was sown shut forever.

There was no one around who remembered enough to answer questions anymore.

~ ~ ~

"Now what?" we wondered. So many old people suddenly were gone. They had been stashed away in nursing homes, hidden away and forgotten like those old wooden clothes pins in their corner kitchen drawers. The old people had the answers. I know they did.

The enemy knew they knew, too. Stashing them away and canceling them wasn't enough, they would have to kill them.

The government blamed their deaths on a plague of sorts. Men in white lab coats told us we all could avoid the same demise if we protected ourselves with a shot of protection right into our arms. The scientific women wore white lab coats, too, punctuated with colorful scarves around their necks, their best shot at looking more feminine, more approachable.

"Run out and protect yourself from certain death!" they told us. "Do it for the greater good!" they told us. "Do your part and the world will be safe!" they told us.

Indeed, your old aunties and uncles and the wise man down the hall had the answers. "We have all those answers you didn't have time to ask us back then," they whispered to us in our memories of them.

The ones remaining silently pleaded with us from darkened corridors, "We will tell you the Truth. There's still time for you to learn."

The enemy prattled on, "Trust us," they said. "Trust the science," they said.

Who were we to listen to? Ancient old talking bones or the smart ones clad in sterile white paper coats clinging onto clipboards, pens in hand?

We saw the refrigerator trucks parked outside the nursing homes. It was wintertime. The ground was frozen. There were so many dead bodies. They showed the workers loading the bodies into the trucks on television, so everyone knew it was real, right?

Frozen in the winter of fear, we knew everyone's mother and father were suddenly in danger of dying, too. We watched as the ancient aunts, the gray-haired uncles, and the elderly grandparents were being unceremoniously stacked into the trucks. We could see the white sheets over their bodies as they were carried out of the nursing homes. The ice picks could not chip the ground fast enough to bury them all.

"We will tell you what to do," they said. "Don't be afraid," they told us. "There's still time for you to learn. Trust us," they said. "We will help you get through this," they said. "Here's a donut," they offered.

"Trust the science," they said.

"Hold your arm still."

~ ~ ~

The plague seemed to be fast-moving, spreading over all the lands of the earth in a flash of light. The television told us the story. Every news channel said the exact same thing. This did not seem odd to most of the people. After all, they had grown up watching *Gilligan's Island* and *Leave It to Beaver* on it. The television had brought us mindless entertainment, and it brought us the important news of the day. *Talking heads chirping the truth, right?*

Back in 1963, Walter Cronkite's gravelly, recognizable voice would deliver the daily events around dinnertime on CBS, always ending his news show with this nightly sign-off: "And that's the way it is." No one questioned it. Why would they?

My parents' generation trusted Walter. Watching the evening news became part of nearly every family's routine after a family dinner of pot roast, carrots and apple pie. Cronkite's signature sign-off, "And that's the way it is," landed directly in our brains through the television box. Everyone trusted him. Why would he lie to us?

~ ~ ~

So many people were lost. They had stopped thinking. Even more had stopped praying. There were only a handful of ears that heard, eyes that saw.

Computers cell phones rabbit ears tinfoil television tell-a-vision programming.

Dazed.

Critical thinking became a crime against humanity. If you did not join the thoughtless wave for "the greater good," then you were deficient. Deficiently defiant and silenced.

Censored.

Useless.

At least to The State.

PART ONE

What It Was Like

And God saw all that He had made, and behold, it was very good.
And there was evening and there was morning, the sixth day.

Genesis 1:31

Chapter One
Creation

Purpose, Purity, Goodness, and Perfection

Look at God's magnificent creation! His glorious Breath of Life. He's designed us in His own image and likeness (Genesis 1:26).

Our Creator set the stage for His highest and most beloved creation, mankind. He created the heavens and the earth, designing gorgeous surroundings with a perfect environment for us to inhabit. He called the light "day" and the dark "night." He created dry land, the seas, the plants and the trees. Then, God made the sun, the moon, the stars, and all of the creatures that inhabit the sea and walk on the land.

On the sixth day of creation, God designed human life in His own image and likeness (Genesis 1:26). In the Garden of Eden, God created the man named Adam and the woman named Eve; and He told them, "Be fruitful and multiply, fill the earth, and subdue it; and rule over the fish of the sea and over the birds of the sky and over every living thing that moves on the earth" (Genesis 1:28).

Then, God generously gave them every plant yielding seed on the surface of all the earth, and every tree which has fruit yielding seed for food. He gave them every green plant for food, "and it was so" (Genesis 1:29-30).

God liked what He created on earth so much (Genesis 1:31), He decided to make a home for Himself there.

> Being made in the image and likeness of God (Genesis 1:27), human beings have the ability to know God and therefore love Him, worship Him, serve Him, and fellowship with Him. God did not create human beings because He needed them. As God, He needs nothing. In all eternity past, He felt no loneliness, so He was not looking for a "friend." He loves us, but this is not the same as needing us. If we had never existed, God would still be God—the unchanging One (Malachi 3:6). The I AM (Exodus 3:14) was never dissatisfied with His own

eternal existence. When He made the universe, He did what pleased Himself, and since God is perfect, His action was perfect. "It was very good" (Genesis 1:31). (https://www.gotquestions.org/why-did-God-create-us.html)

Since God had gifted humanity free will, the ability to decide one's own fate, He recognized there was the possibility that they might rebel against Him. God purposefully created humans with the ability to think and experience a full range of emotions. God was not interested in fellowship with emotionless robots who could not engage in creative thought.

Although it is difficult to define "free will," at a minimum it would mean the ability to make a decision free from coercion and threat.

> If human beings were a product of evolution with no intelligent design involved, then the neural process that is consciousness could possibly be re-created in a robot. However, this is not the case. Genesis 1:27 tells us, "God created man in His own image."

> Mankind did not evolve from simpler life-forms over billions of years. We were designed by God in His image and likeness. Therefore, the human mind is not something a human being could ever replicate. It was designed by an omniscient Creator, and we simply do not have His blueprint.

> What makes a person a person? Job 32:8 says, "But there is a spirit in man, and the breath of the Almighty gives him understanding." God has a [*sic*] placed a spirit in us that makes us human. It's what allows us to think abstractly, create art and music, and appreciate beauty. If God were to take this spirit out of us, we would be like animals.

> Even if people were able to recreate the functions of a human brain in a robot, it would not be alive and conscious because it would not have the spirit in man.

It would not have the spiritual potential to be a child in the family of God. (https://lifehopeandtruth.com/life/blog/why-robots-will-never-be-human/)

Created in God's own image and likeness, mankind was born with creative thought and corresponding emotion:

Being created for God's pleasure does not mean humanity was made to entertain God or provide Him with amusement. God is a creative Being, and it gives Him pleasure to create. God is a personal Being, and it gives Him pleasure to have other beings He can have a genuine relationship with. (https://www.gotquestions.org/why-did-God-create-us.html)

"Human free will is manifested in the fact that, throughout Scripture, God gives us choices and calls on us to choose the way he knows is best." (https://reknew.org/2018/12/where-is-human-free-will-in-the-bible/)

At first it might seem that if God created all things, then evil must have been created by God. However, evil is not a "thing" like a rock or electricity. You cannot have a jar of evil. Evil has no existence of its own; it is really the absence of good. For example, holes are real but they only exist in something else. We call the absence of dirt a hole, but it cannot be separated from the dirt. So, when God created, it is true that all He created was good. One of the good things God made was creatures who had the freedom to choose good. In order to have a real choice, God had to allow there to be something besides good to choose. So, God allowed these free angels and humans to choose good or reject good (evil). (https://www.gotquestions.org/did-God-create-evil.html)

The Bible teaches us that humans possess free will and are capable of choosing to do evil. In the first chapter of the Bible God actually commands mankind to be fruitful and exert dominion over the animal kingdom and the earth (Gen 1:26). The very fact that God commands us to carry out his will acknowledges that we are not forced to carry out his will. We are able to choose to obey God or to choose not to obey Him.

Henry H. Morris, in *Scientific Creationism* explains,

> The entire universe was designed for man and he was appointed by God to exercise dominion over it, as God's steward. It was a perfect environment and man was perfectly equipped to manage it. He should, by all reason, have been content and supremely happy, responding in loving thanksgiving to his Creator who had thus endowed him. God, however, did not create man as a mere machine. God's love was voluntary, and for there to be real fellowship man's love also must be voluntary; in fact, an "involuntary love" is a contradiction in terms. Man was endowed with freedom to love or not love, to obey or not obey, as well as with the responsibility to choose. The history of over 6,000 years of strife and suffering, crime and war, decay and death, is proof enough that he chose wrongly.
>
> Sin came into the world when man first doubted, then rejected, the Word of God in the garden of Eden. And death came into the world when sin came into the world. (Morris, 1974, p. 211)
>
> We were intricately created purposefully in His image. "For you created my inmost being; you knit me together in my mother's womb. I praise you because I am fearfully and wonderfully made" (Psalm 139:13-14).

Author Lee Strobel investigated scientific evidence that points toward God creating us, and he wrote of it in his book, *The Case for a Creator*. He found,

For more than fifty years, as scientists have studied the six feet of DNA that's tightly coiled inside every one of our body's one hundred trillion cells, they have marveled at how it provides the genetic information necessary to create all of the proteins out of which our bodies are built. In fact, each one of the thirty thousand genes that are embedded in our twenty-three pairs of chromosomes can yield as many as 20,500 different kinds of proteins.

The astounding capacity of microscopic DNA to harbor this mountain of information, carefully spelled out in a four-letter chemical alphabet, "vastly exceeds that of any other known system," said geneticist Michael Denton.

In fact, he said the information needed to build the proteins for all the species of organisms that ever lived, a number estimated to be approximately one thousand million "could be held in a teaspoon and there would still be room left for all the information in every book ever written." (Strobel, 2004, pp. 231, 232)

Fearfully and wonderfully created, indeed, with a Creator who gave us everything we need to thrive.

Chapter Two

Everything We Needed to Survive

Nourishment, Dominion, and Perfect Balance

As our loving Creator, perfect Father, and omnipotent giver of life, God provided everything, every single thing, we would need to sustain our lives. He created us to thrive and enjoy our lifetime on earth. He generously filled the gardens with delicious fruits and vegetables and herbs.

Genesis 1:27 states, "God created man in his own image." This scriptural passage does not literally mean God is in human form, but rather, that He created humans in the image of Himself in their moral, spiritual, and intellectual nature.

Since God created mankind in His image and likeness, each person has been guaranteed inherent value by Him. God clearly separated humankind from the life He created in animals and plants. Created in His image, God tells us human worth is not based on race, ethnicity, economic status, social standing, or physical beauty. Hence, the image and likeness of God disallows prejudice of any kind.

> Starting with Adam and Eve, "God reproduces and lives out His image in millions of ordinary people like us. It is a supreme mystery. We are called to bear that image as a Body because any one of us taken individually would present an incomplete image, one partly false and always distorted, like a single glass chip hacked from a mirror. But collectively, in all our diversity, we can come together as a community of believers to restore the image of God in the world." (Brand & Yancey, 1984, p. 40)

Co-authors Philip Yancey and the late Dr. Paul Brand, collaborated in writing a beautiful book, *In the Likeness of God*, metaphorically using the human body both physically and spiritually to describe the Body of Christ as His church on earth, they discussed how God designed us in His image and likeness.

Dr. Brand shared this personal story with us:

> Genesis 2 adds more detail: "And the Lord God formed man from the dust on the ground and breathed into his nostrils the breath of life, and man became a living being (v. 7).

> When I heard that verse as a child, I imagined Adam laying on the ground, perfectly formed but not yet alive, with God leaning over him and performing a sort of mouth-to-mouth resuscitation. Now I picture that scene differently. I assume that Adam was already biologically alive, the other animals needed no special puff of oxygen, nitrogen and carbon dioxide to start them breathing, so why should man? The breath of God now symbolizes for me a spiritual reality. I see Adam as alive, but possessing only animal vitality. Then God breathes into him a new spirit, and infills him with God's own image. Adam becomes a living soul, not just a living body. God's image is not an arrangement of skin cells or a physical shape, but rather an in-breathed spirit.

> This single act of special creation, God breathing into man "the breath of life," distinguished humanity from all other creatures.

> We are made in the image of God. For us, the shell of skin and muscles and bones serves as a vessel, a repository for God's image. We can comprehend and even convey something of the Creator. Our cellular constructions and proteins arranged by DNA can become temples of the Holy Spirit. We are not "mere mortals." We are, all of us, immortals. (Brand & Yancey, 1980, p. 241)

Thus, as the temples of His Holy Spirit, God created the highest and best resources for physical nourishment in food. He gave us clean, pure air to breathe, and provided fresh water for us to drink. He loved us so completely, created us so perfectly, that He made the perfect atmosphere for us to live in, with splendid surroundings around us to see, to fill our hearts with joy and contentment.

God, in His magnificent wisdom and pure love, created mankind skillfully with a perfect balance of Soul, Spirit and Physical Body.

> The three aspects of man: the spirit, the soul, and the body. Body: soma (Greek): the lowest part of man, the physical man, the fleshly or natural man. Soul: nephesh (Hebrew), psyche (Greek): inner nature or man, the person or one's self. Includes the mental, emotional, sensual, and passionate. Soul also refers to the life one has as a person. The soul or life is in the blood. Spirit: ruah (Hebrew), pneuma (Greek): wind, force, or breath. Also rendered as breath: neshamah' (Hebrew). References for above definitions: Unger's Bible Dictionary; Webster's Bible Dictionary; Hayford's Bible Handbook. (https://earlychristianbeliefs.org/the-spirit-soul-body)

Hence, "Now may the God of peace Himself sanctify you entirely; and may your spirit and soul and body be preserved complete, without blame at the coming of our Lord Jesus Christ" (1 Thessalonians 5:23).

While God gave us dominion over the animals (Gen 1:26), we are reminded that God told us to be good stewards of His created earth. God's command for mankind to subdue. His earthly creation was part of God's blessing on mankind. Created in the image of God, Adam and Eve were supposed to use the earth's vast resources in the service of both God and themselves. Of course, God would proclaim this, since only humans, not the animals or the birds or the fish, were created in God's image.

New Zealand-born Christian minister and evangelist Ray Comfort says this is in his booklet, *Scientific Facts in the Bible*:

The Bible tells us that animals are created "without understanding." We are made in God's "image." We aren't merely a higher form of species on the evolutionary scale. As human beings, we are aware of our "being." God is "I AM," and we know that "we are." We have an understanding that we exist. Among other unique characteristics, we have an innate ability to appreciate God's creation. What animal gazes with awe at a sunset, or at the magnificence of the Grand Canyon? What animal obtains joy from the sounds of music or takes time to form itself into an orchestra to create and harmonize music? We are moral human beings. What animal among the beasts sets up court systems and apportions justice to its fellow creatures? (Comfort, 2001, pp. 28-29)

"For You created my innermost parts; You wove me in my mother's womb. I will give thanks to You, because I am awesomely and wonderfully made; Wonderful are Your works, And my soul knows it very well" (Psalm 139:13-14).

Wonder with me! How could we, created in the image and likeness of God, choose to sin, to rebel against the One Who loves us the most, right from the start? How can that be? God's creation was so perfect, He had breathed His Holy Spirit into us, that precious breath of life, and had given us everything we could possibly need.

Chapter Three
Perfect Health

Absence of Pain, Absence of Disease,
No Need for Medicines

God had given us life, breathed into us His Holy Spirit, gifted us with precious free will, provided perfect foods for nourishment, and He gave to us His perfect love from the very moment He created us.

Mankind knew only complete love; God had provided satisfaction for every one of humankind's needs, wants, and desires.

Before there was time, before there was space, when God was all that existed, a brilliant plot was wrapping itself around a grace-full idea. These passionate ideas and plans were being formed in the mind of the Creator and cast a shadow over all of His beloved creation: *The shadow of His presence.*

The imaginations creating the story were in harmony with the love flowing out of the Father's heart. Stimulating the thinking in His mind were the powerful passions stirring in His heart. The thoughts in His mind were eventually translated into words, words that would form the outline of an incredible plan. In the beginning the Scriptures tell us, was the Word. The Word was the full expression of the thoughts of this magnificent Maker. But before a word could exist, there had to be thoughts, conceived from an inspired idea.

Whatever God thinks, is. Father has the power to transform thought into visible reality. His thoughts were gathering themselves together in an orderly and passionate form, ready to be displayed in a glorious manifestation of heavenly magnitude: *all made possible by the Image-Maker.*

The divine idea was magnificent in the breadth of its detail and yet so intimate in the passion of its purpose. Before the divine purpose was manifested in creation it was first conceived in the mind of the Maker. Only a

God of love could conceive of a plan so wonderful, so beautiful, yet so mysterious. (Milam, 2003, pp. 29-30)

"The Lord God planted a garden toward the east, in Eden; and there He placed the man whom He had formed" (Genesis 2:8). God had created man and gave him a home, a model for all future homes, filled with love, freedom, acceptance, creativity, companionship and God's peace. In His marvelous plan, homes would become nations, and nations would reflect the glory of that first home.

"Then the LORD God took the man and put him in the Garden of Eden to cultivate it and tend it" (Genesis 2:15).

> The garden created by the Father was placed under the custodial care of Adam. God placed Adam in the garden to be a creator just like Father. Work was part of God's original purpose for man, but there was perfect order to that work. If the order were violated it would disturb the inner peace of man and have disastrous consequences.

> This was the order: God worked and then He rested, and man begins his work in the realm of Father's rest. Man's first day begins in the rest of God. In that rest he, too, is able to work effectively and creatively. Man must never violate this arrangement. If he does not do his work in the rest of God, then creativity is adversely affected, peace is disrupted, and man's work turns into sweat. There was no sweat in the garden.

> God's world was the source of Adam's creative work in the garden. Man was created to become a creator like his Maker. He would express that creative ability by nurturing the world given to him by Father. Man did not have the ability to create from nothingness like his Father, but he was given a mind and a heart to create powerful and wonderful things from the material supplied by the Creator. (Milam, p. 54, 55)

There was no sweat, no disease, no suffering:

> The Garden of Eden was the perfect environment
> for humans to live in. The climate would have been
> finely tuned to be perfect for humans to live without
> clothing—it would not have been too cold (requiring
> covering) or too warm (resulting in heat stroke or heat
> exhaustion).
>
> The garden was filled with vegetation that was designed
> to provide perfect nutrition (verse 16) for impeccable
> human health. At this time, all animals were tame and
> designed to live at peace with human beings. Adam was
> given the task of naming all the animals (verses 19-20).
> Adam's regular job was to "tend and keep" the garden
> (verse 15).
>
> This garden represented perfect *peace* and *safety* for
> the first human beings. There was no danger, worry,
> violence, sickness or stress. (https://lifehopeandtruth.
> com/bible/blog/god-places-man-in-the-garden-of-
> eden/)

There was a flawless relationship with restorative love at the core:

> God created all things and had a flawless relationship
> with Adam and Eve in the beginning. Everything is
> perfect. Adam and Eve have never heard of cancer,
> murder, heartbreak or pain. They live in unbroken
> fellowship with God and all things. Genesis 3 tells
> us that God walks in the Garden of Eden and speaks
> directly to Adam and Eve. It's hard for us to imagine
> what it is like without arguments, sickness, disease, job
> loss or food insecurity. Everything in Eden functioned
> perfectly through God's creativity, generosity and
> friendship.
>
> But Adam and Eve defy God and eat fruit from
> the forbidden tree. They hide from God knowing
> consequences are coming—and we have been hiding

ever since. Fellowship with God is broken and lost for them and all humanity. The primary consequence is losing the perfect presence of God. They are driven out of Eden and cherubim are placed at the entrance to guard the gate.

Fortunately, this isn't the end. God desires to reclaim his perfect creation and fix what is broken. He desires to restore his presence among people. The Bible shares story after story demonstrating God's plan of restoration. He dwells among the Israelites, sends his son and promises to restore all things. God promises to fix what's broken and once again dwell among his people.

(https://www.beyondtheweekend.org/2021/11/30/november-30-the-garden/)

There is an interesting aspect we simply cannot ignore: Because of God's gift of free will, Adam and Eve could have attained the knowledge of good and evil without ever taking a bite of the fruit from the forbidden tree.

Looking closely at the Words of God, we realize the divinely inspired Bible begins and ends with a garden. The garden becomes a metaphor for a sacred space of both communion and cultivation.

"In the beginning God created..." (Gen. 1:1). God speaks the world into existence. Everything is made out of nothing. First there is silence, stillness, nothing. Then the divine creative word is uttered, the curtain is opened, and a chorus of comets and quasars, seas and volcanoes, and oaks and toads comes forth. He makes a wonderfully diverse biological *community*. God is a community, Father, Son, and Holy Spirit, and we, too, are communal by nature, built to live together in harmony. *Eden is a community garden.*

God calls creation "good" (Gen. 1:31). Material creation is affirmed. The Creator cares about our physical well-being, as well as our spiritual state. He is the God of soil and skin, as well as souls. The creation is characterized by shalom and justice, well-being and harmony; things are the way they are supposed to be. There is no scarcity, only abundance for everyone. With no lack, no conflict, and no pain, *Eden is a peaceful garden.*

In this garden, there is perfect communion between male and female, humans and other creatures, God and all his creation. God walks in the cool of the garden. He relocates from heaven to walk with his people and creation. But there is a unique communion between God and humanity. A relationship has begun, humanity is made in God's image, demonstrated by God's communication to the first pair: "Do not eat..." The garden models this communion between human and divine. *Eden is a lover's garden.*

Since the Creator weaves human creatures in his own image, they, too, are designed for creative work. This is a garden, not a wilderness. God is the first gardener, cultivating it to make it blossom. Cultivate means "tillage; improvement; increase of fertility; the bestowing of labor and care upon a plant, so as to *develop* and improve its qualities." God *develops* his creational community. God may be the first gardener, but then *humanity* is called to cultivate the earth and "to work the ground" (Gen. 2:5). Fruitful labor is part of God's plan, welfare is not. *Eden is a cultivated garden.* (https://inallthings.org/between-two-gardens/)

Truly, God gave mankind His perfect love from the very moment He created us. He gave us the work of going forth, being fruitful and multiplying, filling His gorgeous creation.

Chapter Four
Man and Woman

Pro-Creation and Pro-Life

We know from Genesis 1 and Genesis 2 how the creation of male and female are a part of God's deliberate design for humanity.

> Genesis 1:27 conveys an undeniable connection between "the image of God" and the ontological categories of male and female. This verse consists of three lines of poetry, with the second and third lines structured in parallel, communicating a correlation between God's image and "male and female."
>
> So, God created man in his own image,
>
> in the image of God he created him;
>
> male and female he created them.
>
> Being created in the image of God and being male or female are essential to being human. Sex (male and female) is not simply biological or genetic, just as being human is not simply biological or genetic. *Sex is first and foremost a spiritual and ontological reality created by God.* Being male or female cannot be changed by human hands; sex is a category of God's handiwork, his original and everlasting design. (https://www. desiringgod.org/articles/he-made-them-male-and-female)

The creation of two sexes is indisputable:

> The Bible knows no other gender categories besides male and female. While men and women in Scripture may express their masculinity and femininity in a wonderful diversity of ways, Scripture still operates with the binary categories of men and women. You are one or the other. The anomaly of intersex individuals does not undermine the creational design, but rather gives another example of creational "groaning" and

the "not the way they are supposed to be" realities of a
fallen world. Likewise, the eunuchs in Matthew 19 do
not refer to sexless persons, but to men who were born
without the ability to procreate or who were castrated,
likely for a royal court (for more on the challenge of
intersex, and the question of eunuchs, see Denny Burk,
What Is the Meaning of Sex? 169-183).

Far from being a mere cultural construct, God depicts
the existence of a man and a woman as essential to
his creational plan. The two are neither identical nor
interchangeable. But when the woman, who was taken
out of man, joins again with the man in sexual union,
the two become one flesh (Gen. 1:23-24). Dividing the
human race into two genders, male and female – one or
the other, not both, and not one then the other – is not
the invention of Victorian prudes or patriarchal oafs. It
was God's idea.

As much as contemporary academia says otherwise,
the Bible believes in the organic unity of biological
sex and gender identity. This is why male and female
are (uniquely) the type of pair that can reproduce
(Gen. 1:28; 2:20). It's why homosexuality–a man
lying with a man and a woman with a woman (Lev.
18:22)–is wrong. It's why the apostle Paul can speak of
homosexual partnerships as deviating from the natural
relations or natural function of male-female sexual
intercourse (Rom. 1:26-27). In each instance, the
argument only works if there is an assumed equivalence
between the biology of sexual difference and the
corresponding identities of male and female.

(https://www.thegospelcoalition.org/blogs/
kevin-deyoung/what-does-the-bible-say-about-
transgenderism/)

While the expectations for the roles of male and female may be
shaped by a society's cultural norms, God's Word tells us each sex

is distinct in their role in His creative process. This distinction of calling each as biblical manhood and womanhood, is not necessarily acknowledged in the secular world.

> In the creation account, God creates the woman to be the man's "helper fit for him" (Genesis 2:18). The word *helper* (Hebrew *'ezer*) does not denote a person of lesser worth or value. In fact, *'ezer* occurs 21 times in the Old Testament, and 16 of these refer to God as Israel's help.
>
> Transgenderism is not exclusively a battle for what is male and female, but rather a battle for what is true and real.
>
> "Fit for him" (*kenegdo*) communicates complementarity, both similarity and dissimilarity. Adam and Eve are both alike as human beings and also not alike as male and female. God intends for the woman to complement and not duplicate the man. This difference of calling is God's design from the beginning.
>
> The apostle Paul exhorts husbands to love their wives "as Christ loved the church and gave himself up for her" (Ephesians 5:25) and wives to submit to their husbands "as the church submits to Christ" (Ephesians 5:24). These distinct callings are vital in marriage, the church, and other realms as well. (https://www.desiringgod.org/articles/he-made-them-male-and-female)

God's world does not change, His creation does not come up for "renewal" or an "upgrade" unless He says so.

> In the increasingly brainwashed world we live in, it is incredibly refreshing when experts are willing to speak the politically incorrect truth. In Thursday's edition of the *Wall Street Journal*, biologists Colin M. Wright and

Emma N. Hilton provide extensive commentary on the transgender fad and the notion of gender fluidity.

With the phenomenon of some men saying they "identify" as women and some women saying they "identify" as men, or any "gender identity" combination therein, "we see a dangerous and anti-scientific trend toward the outright denial of biological sex," state the biologists Wright and Hilton.

This notion that there is a sex "spectrum," where people can choose "to identify as male or female," regardless of their anatomy, is irrational and has "no basis in reality," say the biologists. "It is false at every conceivable scale of resolution."

As they explain, "In humans, as in most animals or plants, an organism's biological sex corresponds to one of two distinct types of reproductive anatomy that develop for the production of small or large sex cells—sperm and eggs, respectively—and associated biological functions in sexual reproduction."

"In humans, reproductive anatomy is unambiguously male or female at birth more than 99.98% of the time," they write. "The evolutionary function of these two anatomies is to aid in reproduction via the fusion of sperm and ova."

"No third type of sex cell exists in humans, and therefore there is no sex 'spectrum' or additional sexes beyond male and female," state the biologists. "Sex *is* binary."

Furthermore, "the existence of only two sexes does not mean sex is never ambiguous," write Hilton and Wright. "But intersex individuals are extremely rare, and they are neither a third sex nor proof that sex is a 'spectrum' or a 'social construct.'"

What does the science say? In short, it says that
are only two genders: male and female. (https://
pjmedia.com/culture/matt-margolis/2020/02/15/
science-says-there-are-only-two-genders-no-gender-
spectrum-n379108)

There is absolutely no wiggle-room on this one, either. In order to go forth and multiply,

> God created man in His own image, in the image of
> God He created him; male and female He created them.
> God blessed them; and God said to them, "Be fruitful
> and multiply, and fill the earth, and subdue it; and rule
> over the fish of the sea and over the birds of the sky
> and over every living thing that moves on the earth"
> (Genesis 1:27-28).

Pro-creation, procreation, becomes the cornerstone in God's blueprint for Creation.

Chapter Five
The Firmament

The Dome of the Divine

The heavens tell of the glory of God;
And their expanse declares the work of His hands.
Psalm 19:1

Then God said,
"Let there be an expanse in the midst of the waters,
and let it separate the waters from the waters."
God made the expanse, and separated the waters
that were below the expanse from the waters
that were above the expanse; and it was so.
God called the expanse "heaven."
And there was evening and there was morning, a second day.
Genesis 1:6-8

The firmament was created by God on the second day; there were "waters above the firmament" (Genesis 1:7).

It would efficiently filtering [*sic*] harmful radiation from space, markedly reducing the rate of somatic mutations in living cells, and, as a consequence, drastically decreasing the rate of aging and death." (Morris, 1974, p. 211)

This would be one of the reasons mankind was able to live for hundreds of years. They were living in a protected, tropical paradise.

Later, the firmament (canopy over the earth) collapsed in the form of rain (the "windows of heaven" in Genesis 7:11), contributing to the flood water in the days of Noah, and resulting in the dramatic drop-off in the longevity of life after the deluge. Before the flood, the average lifespan of a person was 900 years.

The existence of a "firmament" has been one of the greatest puzzles concerning the Creation account, mostly because of its Hebrew definition:

> רָקִיעַ raqiya` raw-kee'-ah
>
> from 7554; properly, an expanse, i.e., the firmament or (apparently) visible arch of the sky: firmament. (https://www.kjvbible.org/firmament.html)

We are left to wonder, *Is it an arch? Is it a canopy? Does it still exist?*

> And God said, "Let there be lights in the firmament of the heaven to divide the day from the night; and let them be for signs, and for seasons, and for days, and years: And let them be for lights in the firmament of the heaven to give light to the earth: and it was so. And God made two great lights; the greater light to rule the day, and the lesser light to rule the night: He made the stars also. (Genesis 1:14-16 KJV)

Dr. Oren Fass described his "encounter with the firmament" this way,

> Of all the vexing problems modern cosmology poses for the first chapter of Genesis, such as the insufficient biblical timeline of 6 days (as opposed to billions of years) until the appearance of humans, or vegetative bloom before the sun and photosynthesis, the most acute for me is God's creation of the firmament (עיקר; *rakia*) on the second day.

Fass continues,

> If you are unfamiliar with the firmament, then imagine for a moment the horizon, where the earth appears to meet with the sky. Only try to picture it as a connecting point between two solids: a flat plate like earth, and a rigid dome like an upside down bowl that vaults it, blue as ocean, from the vast stores of water it contains. This is what the Bible is describing when it refers to עיְקְרָה, traditionally rendered in English Bibles as "the firmament" (from the Latin firmamentum meaning "support").
>
> If you can entertain this notion, and feel yourself underneath this massive curved wall of heaven, straining under the weight of the rainwater it holds back, then you are living on the earth our sages knew, for this is the world, the universe, of which the Bible conceived:
>
> [In Genesis 1:6-8,] God said, "Let there be a firmament in the midst of the water, that it may separate water from water." God made the firmament, and it separated the water which was below the firmament from the water which was above the firmament. And it was so. God called the firmament Sky...

The idea of a firmament is entirely contradictory
to modern planetary science; yet there God is, in
our Torah, spending all of creation day number two
fashioning it. (https://www.thetorah.com/article/my-
encounter-with-the-firmament)

More Torah experts weigh in on the subject:

Why is the sky blue during the daytime? The scientific
answer is that molecules of air in the atmosphere
scatter blue light from the sun. At night, when the
earth is facing away from the sun, there is no light to
scatter and the sky is black. The scattering of light
by the atmosphere is called the Tyndall effect, named
after the scientist John Tyndall who first suggested this
mechanism in 1859.

But the ancient cosmologist was living in a different
world than Tyndall. In his conception, the earth is the
center of the universe, and the sun, moon and stars
travel above it, in the firmament. When this ancient
cosmologist asked himself why the day-time sky is blue,
his answer was because there is light in the heavenly
water above the firmament. As he would have seen from
earth, water is blue and thus when the light enters the
water, the sky looks blue. When the light leaves the
water and darkness creeps in, it is black.

The light and darkness in this conception should be
pictured as diffuse physical substances that permeate
the waters of the heavens. The sun, in this conception,
is a totally separate light. Richard Elliott Friedman, in
his gloss on v. 15, describes this view in the following
manner:

Note that daylight is not understood here to derive
from the sun. The text understands the light that
surrounds us in the daytime to be an independent

creation of God, which has already taken place on the first day. The sun, moon, and stars are understood here to be light sources—like a lamp or torch, only stronger. Their purpose is also to be markers of time: days, years, appointed occasions. [See Richard Elliott Friedman, *Commentary on the Torah* (San Francisco: Harper, 2001)] (https://www.thetorah.com/article/if-the-sun-is-created-on-day-4-what-is-the-light-on-day-1

Moshe Weinfeld, in his commentary on Genesis (1:3), offers the same overall reading:

> The light is not dependent on the lights created on the fourth day, in accordance with the viewpoint popular during that period that light and darkness are independent entities that exist in hidden places [of the heavens] dedicated to them (Job 39:19-20). Weinfeld's commentary is part of the revised version of the Samuel Gordon's commentary, reprinted by Galil B.D. Nagar ltd. [*sic*] in 1992.

The text to which Weinfeld calls the readers' attention is God's speech to Job:

> Job 38:12 Have you ever commanded the day to break, assigned the dawn its place... 38:18 Have you surveyed the expanses of the earth? If you know of these - tell Me. 38:19 Which path leads to where light dwells, and where is the place of darkness, 38:20 That you may take it to its domain and know the way to its home?

> God here asks Job whether he knows where light and darkness are stored, implying that these two substances are discrete entities in and of themselves. When one is spread out in the heavens, the other is sitting in its appointed spot awaiting its turn. (https://www.thetorah.com/article/if-the-sun-is-created-on-day-4-what-is-the-light-on-day-1)

Genesis 1:16 describes the creation of the sun and moon this way: "God made the two great lights, the greater light to govern the day, and the lesser light to govern the night; He made the stars also."

The Canopy, the Light, the Dark, Food, Beauty, Creative Work. God's creation included everything we needed to survive, to thrive and to be happy.

Chapter Six

Enter the Serpent

The Enemy Appears

Despite the abundance of foods available literally at their fingertips, a serpent, the ultimate antagonist, tempted Eve with the one thing God had forbidden them to eat. Twining itself seductively around the branches of a tree, it beckoned her.

> Genesis chapter 3 of the Bible recounts the story of Adam, the first man God created, and the woman God formed from one of Adam's ribs. They lived piously in the Garden of Eden until the serpent, craftier than the other animals, led the woman into temptation. The serpent said, "Did God actually say 'You shall not eat of any tree in the garden? [*sic*]'" The woman answered, "We may eat of the fruit of the trees in the garden, but God said, 'You shall not eat of the fruit of the tree that is in the midst of the garden, neither shall you touch it, lest you die.'" The serpent replied, "You will not surely die. For God knows that when you eat of it your eyes will be opened, and you will be like God, knowing good and evil." Since the woman sought wisdom, she ate the fruit of the tree, and gave some to Adam to eat too. "Then the eyes of both of them were opened, and they knew that they were naked."

> When God came into the garden, they hid from him. He noticed that they had eaten the fruit of the tree of knowledge, and turned them out of Paradise. "To Adam he said, 'Because you have listened to the voice of your wife and have eaten of the tree of which I commanded you, 'You shall not eat of it', cursed is the ground because of you; in pain you shall eat of it all the days of your life; thorns and thistles it shall bring forth for you; and you shall eat the plants of the field. By the sweat of your face you shall eat bread, till you return to the ground, for out of it you were taken; for you are

dust and to dust you shall return." After the fall, Adam named his wife Eve (which means 'life' in Hebrew), as the mother of all living, the progenitrix of all human beings.

Theology refers to this incident as the 'fall of man' as, against God's will, he ate the fruit that allowed him to distinguish good from evil. The Bible does not actually mention an apple, early Christian art depicts the Fall of Man by a fig. Christianity likely introduced the idea of the fruit being an apple, in recollection of the 'apple of paradise' or when the Bible was translated. In Latin, evil is *malum* and an apple is called *malus*. This could have been either a simple mistranslation or a deliberate play on these words." (https://www.alimentarium. org/en/knowledge/eve-and-forbidden-fruit)

There are so many questions arising from the fall of mankind found in Genesis. Is the story of Adam and Eve metaphorical for the fall of humanity or was there truly a garden and did this event really occur? Was "the Serpent" the only animal that talked in the Garden of Eden? Did Satan turn himself into a serpent or did he simply use the snake to speak through to get to Eve? Is it possible that Satan still speaks audibly through animals, or through people today?

The Society for Old Testament Study, founded in 1917, an academic learned society embracing the Old Testament, and its cognate areas such as Hebrew and other Semitic languages, tells us this:

The name Adam (Hebrew 'adam), means 'man,' in the sense of 'human being', 'person', or, most relevantly, 'humanity' in general. However, it appears to be used in this story to refer only to the male person of the first human couple as representative of humanity. It is not widely realized that the Garden of Eden narrative regularly refers to 'the man' (Hebrew ha'adam) rather than to 'Adam'. Although there are just three places in this narrative where the standard Hebrew (Masoretic) text, with its vowels, makes the word a personal name, in the phrase le'adam "to/for Adam" (Gen 2:20; 3:17-21), this is a matter of a mere vowel point, and it is generally accepted that the word would originally have been read la'adam, 'to/for the man,' especially since the expression 'the man' (ha'adam) continues after these references. It is not until Gen 4:25 that the text refers to Adam as a personal name, presumably because by then there are other men around. Adam also appears as a personal name in the Priestly (P) source genealogy in Gen 5:1, 3-5.

Having been created, the man is placed by God in the Garden of Eden and forbidden to eat from the tree of the knowledge of good and evil. But his wife Eve, subsequently created as Adam's helper, having been formed from one of Adam's ribs, is tempted to do that very thing by the serpent (Satan is a later interpretation). Eve then offers some of the fruit to Adam. As a result they are both said to be conscious of their nakedness, an example of the 'knowledge of good and evil' they have acquired. Various punishments are subsequently inflicted in turn by God on the serpent, Eve, and Adam, and Adam and Eve are finally cast out of the garden, thereby denying them access to the tree of life, whose fruit bestows immortality. However, Adam (along with Eve) does not die on the very same day that the fruit is eaten, contrary to what God had originally threatened. Modern scholars dispute the reason for this; most naturally it was a consequence of God's compassion.

(https://www.sots.ac.uk/)

Even if one supposes Adam was not a singular human entity from whom Eve was fashioned from his rib, Adam nonetheless represents humanity's fall from God's grace.

John Calahan, a retired pastor of a non-denominational church now devoting himself full-time to the on-line teaching ministry has this to say about talking serpents and other demons:

> Some have conjectured that all of the animals in the Garden of Eden were able to talk. However, we cannot prove that since scripture does not tell us. We do not have any eyewitnesses, and there are no other records about animals at that time. We only know that the serpent was able to speak on the occasion when Satan spoke through it.

> Now the serpent was more crafty than any beast of the field which the LORD God had made. "And he said to the woman, "Indeed, has God said, 'You shall not eat from any tree of the garden'?" (Genesis 3:1).

> Scripture reveals that when a demon possesses someone, the demon is able to speak through the person's voice. The demon somehow takes control of the person and speaks using their voice. One such incident is recorded in the gospel of Luke when Jesus was in the city of Capernaum.

> In the synagogue there was a man possessed by the spirit of an unclean demon, and he cried out with a loud voice, "Let us alone! What business do we have with each other, Jesus of Nazareth? Have You come to destroy us? I know who You are the Holy One of God!" (Luke 4:33-34).

> If a demon, unclean spirit, or evil angel can speak through a person whom they possess, can they speak through an animal? Genesis 3:1 indicates that the answer is, "Yes!"

> Demons or unclean spirits still speak through people today. Demons or spirits speak through mediums in séances. This is a common occurrence. However, there are many false mediums today who pretend

to communicate with the dead. Evil spirits have always been capable of speaking through people. Unfortunately, we do not know if demons speak through animals today. We are not aware of any evidence.

The author C. S. Lewis (1898-1963) wrote the Chronicles of Narnia [*sic*]. In this series the author has the animals speak to humans. The story line claims that animals did speak in the ancient days. It is an interesting and powerful thought. The answers to your questions reveal that demons are active, real, and powerful. We would encourage you to have nothing to do with them because God has warned us to have nothing to do with them (Deut. 18:14). Do you know Jesus as your Lord and Savior? Have you believed in Jesus? We encourage you to explore "Searching for God." (https://www.neverthirsty.org/bible-qa/qa-archives/question/was-the-serpent-the-only-animal-that-talked-in-the-garden-of-eden/)

Biblica, the International Bible Society, adds this interesting thought about what happened in the garden of Eden:

> Perhaps the author of Genesis skipped over the part where Eve threw up her hands in surprise and exclaimed, "How are you talking to me? None of the other animals can talk. What's going on here!?!"

> Maybe Eve was so new to the Garden that she had yet to realize none of the other animals could talk.

> Or perhaps talking animals were not all that unusual. It's certainly something to think about.

> Whatever tempted Eve did NOT look like a snake as we think of them today.

> You've undoubtedly seen plenty of illustrations showing Eve being tempted by a slithering snake. Is that an accurate image?

In Genesis 3:14 God said to the serpent, "Because you have done this, cursed are you above all livestock and all wild animals! You will crawl on your belly and you will eat dust all the days of your life."

But if the serpent began life on his belly *after* Eve ate the forbidden fruit, it makes sense that it didn't crawl on its belly *before* the fall. Before the curse, did the serpent walk upright? Did it have legs or even wings? We'll never know until we get to Heaven but it seems safe to say that the common perception of a legless serpent tempting Eve is wrong.

(https://www.biblica.com/articles/7-interesting-things-you-may-not-have-considered-about-the-garden-of-eden/)

The enemy's evil tricks have continued to cause mayhem throughout history. God has created a wonderful world for us to live in; mankind's misuse of His gift of free will has wreaked havoc over and over.

Chapter Seven

The Father of Lies

The Only Way Out

Rebellion.

Indeed, this did happen in the Garden of Eden. We have seen how richly God had blessed Adam and Eve, (Genesis 1:22-28), and how they rebelled (Genesis 3), resulting in the fall of mankind.

Nearly 1,000 years after Adam and Eve's rebellion, sin had plummeted the world into a state of serious debauchery.

The Flood of Noah's day (2348 BC), destroyed the world, reshaped the continents, buried billions of creatures, and laid down the rock layers. It formed huge basins of puddles and changed the landscape of the earth forever.

The flood was God's judgment on man's decision to choose wickedness, and only eight righteous people and two of every kind of land animal were spared aboard Noah's ark. Noah was an obedient servant of God who found favor with God in a sinful world. Noah had built the ark according to God's specifications.

Noah and his family had to stay on the ark for ten months after it stopped raining, waiting for dry land to appear,

> According to the Masoretic Hebrew text, as interpreted literally by fundamentalists, the Flood occurred 1656 years after the creation of Adam. Then Noah was 600 years old, so he would have been born 1056 years after creation.
>
> (https://www.quora.com/How-much-time-passed-in-the-Bible-between-the-time-of-Adam-and-Eve-and-the-time-of-Noah)

Four hundred years after the flood, God chose Abram to be the man to help Him carry out His plan for a home for Himself on earth, complete with His own nation where the people were His.

> Abraham's place in the Bible's portrait gallery is altogether unique and unapproachable. He stands

out as a landmark in the spiritual history of the world. Chosen of God to become the father of a new spiritual race, the file leader of a mighty host, the revelation of God found in him one of its most important epochs. In himself, there was not much to make him worthy of such a distinction. His choice was all of grace. (https://www.biblegateway.com/resources/all-men-bible/Abram-Abraham)

Chapter 12 in the Book of Genesis marks the moment when God decided to make Israel his homeland with the Israelites his chosen people. God knew this would be the place salvation would be offered to mankind through faith in His only Son. Abram's name later was changed to Abraham. Abraham was the first Hebrew patriarch and is revered in Judaism, Christianity and Islam.

God's command to Abram was to go away from his country, his people, and his fathers house. At 75 years old, Abram was middle-aged for his day. He was comfortable in wealth and was married to a woman named Sarai.

God, without explanation or condition, promised Abram that he would have a great nation of his own. Then, God told Abram He would use him to accomplish wonderful things. God told Abram his name would be so great that He would bless people who blessed him and curse those who dishonored him.

Abram answered God with a "yes." Certainly, the promises must have been well beyond anything Abram ever imagined for his life. In response to this command, Abram, Sarai, Abram's nephew Lot, and their hand-picked large troupe of assistants headed into the land of Canaan. That was the territory that one day would become the Promised Land (Genesis 12:7).

The plan did not always go smoothly for Abram and Sarai. They faced famine and entire tribes of cities while unarmed. Abram was tested along the way, failing a few times. Yet, God remained faithful, resulting in the establishment of Israel to have a place on earth for His chosen people.

God had gifted humans free will at the beginning of Creation, opening the door to the probability of mankind choosing to "sin." Therefore, God had to make a way to reconcile humanity to Himself. He accomplished this through Abram and the promises He gave him. Ultimately, God blessed Abram, and changed his name to Abraham.

It was through Abraham's lineage that the Savior of the world would come (Matthew 1; Luke 3). Abraham was the first man chosen by God to have a role in His plan of redemption.

Recall how God blessed Adam and Eve at the beginning of creation (Genesis 1:22-28), and then, and how their disobedience to God resulted in the fall of mankind (Genesis 3). The story of Abram reveals how God blessed His human kind again when He sought restoration and conciliation through the newly-named Abraham and his descendants (Genesis 12:1-3).

The Book of Genesis laid the foundation for all of the history of redemption. God's work of salvation for mankind continued throughout the remainder of the Old Testament and into the New Testament. The covenant between Abraham and God consisted of three separate parts: the promised land, the promise of descendants, and the promise of blessing and redemption.

Ultimately, God's agreements with His children were established to keep His Creation blameless and pure.

Wonder with me! How could mankind misuse free will to the extent of falling so far from God's goodness? How can that be? Where does such evil come from? Let's revisit the Garden for another moment.

Chapter Eight

Temptation

Free Will and the Fall of Man

The Lord God sent Adam and Eve out of the Garden of Eden after their act of disobedience. God then "stationed the cherubim and the flaming sword which turned every direction to guard the way to the tree of life" (Genesis 3:24), ensuring that they would not be able to return to the garden.

Since then, mankind has endured pain, suffering, and heartache in every aspect of our lives, including the pangs of childbirth and the struggle to provide for our families. The act of disobedience, the falling into the state of sin, is referred to as the fall of man because Adam's sin did not just apply to him but to every human being who would live in this world.

Genesis 2:16-17 says, "The LORD God commanded the man, saying, "From any tree of the garden you may freely eat; but from the tree of the knowledge of good and evil you shall not eat, for on the day that you eat from it you will certainly die." The presence of the tree was important because Adam was gifted with free will; so therefore, there would have to be a choice for him to make a decision, presenting an opportunity to decide to go against God's command.

If a command is not present, if there is nothing forbidden, then there cannot be a rebellious decision. It's not the choice that causes a problem, it is the personal responsibility attached to the decision one makes regarding the presented choice. God asks that our decisions be rooted in love and obedience toward Him as our generous Creator. "On the day that you eat of it you shall surely die." God made His command clear to Adam, and He also made the consequences for disobedience clear as well.

God created mankind with a physical body, breathed life into him (Spirit), and gave him the gift of free will (Soul) to decide his own eventual fate. A decision against God's command for an individual surely will always result in punishment; conversely, decisions made in alignment with God's commands will result in blessings from Him.

Hence, God is not specifically referring to corporal death (the Body), He is warning of the consequences to the spirit and soul, too.

> Satan, the serpent, the liar, beckons with this deception,

> Now the serpent was more cunning than any animal of the field which the LORD God had made. And he said to the woman, "Has God really said, 'You shall not eat from any tree of the garden'?" The woman said to the serpent, "From the fruit of the trees of the garden we may eat; but from the fruit of the tree which is in the middle of the garden, God has said, 'You shall not eat from it or touch it, or you will die.'" The serpent said to the woman, "You certainly will not die! For God knows that on the day you eat from it your eyes will be opened, and you will become like God, knowing good and evil (Genesis 3:1-5).

> How can we be sure the serpent is Satan?

> Ezekiel 28 tells us Satan, before his fall, was an angel of the highest rank and prominence, even something of a leader of worship in heaven. Isaiah 14 tells us Satan's fall had to do with his desire to be equal to or greater than God, to set his will against God's will.

> We may not understand everything involved in the way Satan used the body of a serpent, but we can know it was true and this is no mere fable. "It is idle to call the narrative of the Fall a mere allegory; one had better say at once that he does not believe the Book... There was a real serpent, as there was a real paradise; there was a real Adam and Eve, who stood at the head of our race, and they really sinned, and our race is really fallen. Believe this (Spurgeon). (https://enduringword.com/bible-commentary/genesis-3/)

God presented the tree as a limitation on Adam and Eve. The tree was a reminder to them that they were not God, that He had full rights to their obedience. Ultimately, they were fully responsible to Him, and to Him alone.

The serpent boldly lied to Eve, telling her, "You will not surely die," urging her to think for herself and forget about what God said. Satan directly challenged Eve to consider God as a liar. Satan tells Eve that she won't die. Satan presents his logical syllogism that, if God lies to her and she does not physically die from eating the fruit, then how can God be good?

Eve doubts God and doubts the consequences of her decision. Satan challenges her to doubt the consequences of sin. After all, if fruit is something good for her, why doesn't God want her to have it? The confusion sets in, the enemy knows he has her attention. After all, the fruit is good and an awful God doesn't want her to have it.

This is Satan's lie to us to this day, that sin is not bad, and God is not good. As a matter of fact, this is all a fairy tale, and God doesn't exist anyway, he tells us. Satan knows death of the flesh is one thing and death of the spirit is completely different.

Satan tells Eve she will be like God and know all good and evil. This final lie to Eve is both treacherous and powerful because he knows that his desire to be equal with God is exactly what got him thrown out of heaven. The serpent is tricking Eve into becoming a god by rebelling against God.

The serpent cunningly did not tell Adam and Eve this truth: Even if they took a bite of the fruit, their bodies would not die, but they would no longer be led by the spirit that originally led them to have communion with God. Satan knew tampering with their soul (free will), would kill their spirit.

> While the Fall of Man changed the course of history,
> it also became the backdrop for the glory of God to
> display his mercy and kindness toward humankind.
> Prior to the Fall of man, God and mankind experienced
> communion and fellowship in a close relationship.
> Humankind's nature was created righteous and
> encouraged to do good, to have a conscious

relationship with God, be introduced to the concept of and to be established in the ways of righteousness and faith. Adam and Eve needed to act on their belief in the righteousness of God. The Fall of Man can be defined as the transition from a state of moral innocence, righteousness, and favor with God to a state of separation and death. The hope that can be found from the Fall of Man is the promised redemption in the person and work of Jesus Christ.

When all a person knows is good, I can see how someone could come in and plant doubts. *"If God was truly good, then why wouldn't he say yes to everything?"* That is at the crux of the serpent's question in Genesis 3. But in God's infinite wisdom, a no is not a reflection of his goodness, but of his desire for us to grow in other areas. By having boundaries placed around the tree [*sic*] of knowledge and life, Adam and Eve were introduced to the concept of obedience by choice. Obedience by choice is one way to display our love and respect for God. We obey God because we love him. We love him because he first loved us. We can trust him because he is good. But when faced with a no, instead of looking at it through the lens that God is good and loves me, we view it through, *"If he loved me, he would let me do and be whatever I want."* But a good parent puts boundaries in place out of loving protection. God's goodness prompts him to do the same.

Even though Adam and Eve gave up their intimate union with the Lord, and caused separation from the Lord, he promised hope. Through God's mercy, grace, and love for humankind he made a way for us to be reunited in that intimate relationship. God promised to send a redeemer, his Son, who would bridge the separation gap between a holy, righteous God and a sinful, human race. When God sacrificed an animal and made them clothes from the skins it was a foreshadow of the way he would save us through the sacrifice of a substitute, the shedding of blood, and the covering of righteousness. When Jesus, The Messiah, came, he shed his blood, took our place, and became our righteousness."

(https://www.crosswalk.com/faith/bible-study/ things-to-know-about-the-fall-of-man.html)

Which brings this question to the forefront: "If our decisions are determined anyway, what does it mean to have free will in the first place?" The answer is self-evident:

We have free will *if our choices are determined by that which we experientially identify with.* I identify with my tastes and preferences—as consciously felt by me—in the sense that I regard them as expressions of myself. My choices are thus free insofar as they are determined by these felt tastes and preferences.

(https://blogs.scientificamerican.com/observations/ yes-free-will-exists/)

Free will is the capacity to determine a personal outcome without the influence of the environment or heredity. The antonym of free will, according to modern psychology, is called "hard determinism," the belief that all our decisions are "caused."

The determinist approach proposes that all behavior has a cause and is thus predictable. Free will is an illusion, and our behavior is governed by internal or external forces over which we have no control.

(https://www.simplypsychology.org/freewill- determinism.html)

Recall how before the fall of Adam, man was sinless. For God "saw everything that he had made, and behold, it was very good" (Genesis

1:31). But mankind also was given the gift of free will, allowing him to be susceptible to the act of sinning. God had warned, "On the day that you eat of it [the tree] you shall surely die" (Genesis 2:17).

Cheerful submission to God's authority is something we struggle with as humans with free will. Let's face it, without discipline, we prefer our own authority, believing our big ideas will somehow be better than our Creator's ideas. It's called pride of self. It's rooted in self-will; the belief we know best what is good for us over anyone or anything else's thinking or ideas.

It's not that we are prevented from doing what we think is best for ourselves.

Free will deems we will prefer our own authority, treasuring our own value above God's authority. Defiant, we do not see God. We only see ourselves. We cannot defer to God's insight and supreme wisdom when we are busy preferring the pleasuring of ourselves and satisfying of our own desires.

The problem is this: We don't always know what is best for us. We come to know how our Creator does, though.

> Spiritual death is best understood as alienation or separation of our souls from God. Sin separates us from God, the source and fountain of spiritual life and light (Ephesians 2:12). The spiritually dead sit in darkness and in the shadow of death (Luke 1:79). Because God is holy and sin is offensive to God, our spiritual death is not an amicable separation, but a hostile one (Romans 8:7-8) Scripture describes the spiritually dead as enemies of God (Romans 5:10). The penalty for sin is death (Romans 3:23), and therefore the spiritually dead are cursed and condemned for failing to keep God's law (Galatians 3:10), and await God's wrath (Romans 2:5). They are, in fact, dead men walking.
>
> To be spiritually dead means to be insensible to the things of God and ignorant of spiritual realities (1

Corinthians 2:14). A spiritually dead person does not love God and cannot please God (Romans 8:8). In fact, they want to please themselves, not God (Philippians 2:21). They may appear to perform good deeds from an external perspective in that their deeds conform to the letter of the law. However, these deeds do not conform to the spirit of the law because they are not motivated by a desire to please and glorify God (1 Corinthians 10:31). The spiritually dead can look beautiful on the outside and inside be filled with death, like whitewashed tombs (Matthew 23:27-28).

(https://www.compellingtruth.org/spiritually-dead.html)

So, where does that leave us? There is temptation everywhere.

Chapter Nine
Our Creator Sees It All

The Point of View

How do we arrive at our personal points of view? Conjecture? Intuition? Persuasion post-presentation of scientific evidence? We know scientific hypotheses are conjectural explanations for phenomena occurring in the natural world, always subject to further testing for proof of existence. It's the first step toward establishing the provable scientific method. Basically, it's an "educated guess" rooted in prior experience and observation:

> Science is a systematic and logical approach to discovering how things in the universe work. It is also the body of knowledge accumulated through the discoveries about all the things in the universe.

> The word "science" is derived from the Latin word "scientia," which means knowledge based on demonstrable and reproducible data, according to the Merriam-Webster dictionary. (https://www. livescience.com/20896-science-scientific-method. html)

A hypothesis is not just "a guess." While an "educated guess" suggests a predictable outcome based on a person's experience and expertise in an area, in developing a scientific hypothesis it is necessary to engage in active observation coupled with extensive background research.

> The basic idea of a hypothesis is that there is no predetermined outcome. For a solution to be termed a scientific hypothesis, it has to be an idea that can be supported or refuted through carefully crafted experimentation or observation. This concept, called falsifiability and testability, was advanced in the mid-20th century by Austrian-British philosopher Karl Popper in his famous book "The Logic of Scientific Discovery" [sic] (Routledge, 1959).

A key function of a hypothesis is to derive predictions about the results of future experiments and then perform those experiments to see whether they support the predictions. (https://www.livescience.com/21490-what-is-a-scientific-hypothesis-definition-of-hypothesis.html)

In other words: An educated guess, trial and error in the form of experimentation, conclusive results supporting predictive evidence.

Mathematical evidence is brought to us in the evidence found in "proofs."

In the simplest of words, "Let's see."

Words. Points of view. Proof.

"Now faith is the certainty of things hoped for, a proof of things not seen" (Hebrews 11:1).

Let's take a look together at the Tower of Babel.

God's point of view vs. Man's point of view often does not coincide. Mankind, in the worldly viewpoint, yearns to be self-sufficient. God says,

> "My grace is sufficient for you, for power is perfected in weakness." Most gladly, therefore, I will rather boast about my weaknesses, so that the power of Christ may dwell in me. Therefore, I delight in weaknesses, in insults, in distresses, in persecutions, in difficulties, in behalf of Christ; for when I am weak, then I am strong (2 Cor 12:9-10).

The story of the Tower of Babel in Chapter 11 of the Book of Genesis is a good example of these opposing views. Here's a brief summary of that story:

> "The descendants of Noah were living in the area of Mesopotamia in Babylon. They settled in a land named Shinar. The population was growing and they all spoke one language. The people decided to build a tall, proud symbol of how great they had made their nation. The

Babylonians wanted a tower that would 'reach to the heavens' so that they could be like God and that they would not need Him ....

God did not like the pride and arrogance in the hearts of the people. God caused the people to suddenly speak different languages so they could not communicate and work together to build the tower. This caused the people to scatter across the land. The tower was named The Tower of Babel because the word Babel means confusion. This story is a powerful reminder of how important it is to obey God's Word and not to think that we can build a successful but godless life on our own!" (https://www.faithwriters.com/article-details.php?id=200587)

As Nimrod began his reign, he and his followers had one overriding goal for their new territory; they wanted to ensure the security of their community by building a prestigious landmark to make a name for themselves. "Then they said, 'Come, let us build ourselves a city, with a tower that reaches to the heavens, so that we may make a name for ourselves; otherwise we will be scattered over the face of the whole earth" (Genesis 11:4).

The structure—a tower made from man-made building materials—would be a symbol of their power and self-sufficiency, and some historians believe that Nimrod had an additional motive for wanting to build the tower of Babel. (https://www.biblestudytools.com/bible-stories/the-tower-of-babel.html)

He also said he would be revenged on God, if he should have a mind to drown the world again; for that he would build a tower too high for the waters to be able to reach! [*sic*] and that he would avenge himself on God for destroying their forefathers!

(https://www.biblestudytools.com/history/flavius-
josephus/antiquities-jews/book-1/chapter-4.html)

The people were working together to build this tall monument
to themselves, steeped in arrogance, in complete opposition toward
God's command to multiply and "fill the earth" (Genesis 9:1). They
joined forces with each other to create a nation for themselves, a place
of communal sovereignty with their own self-sufficiency at the center.

They wanted nothing of God ruling over them. They could rule
themselves, reaching heaven on their own terms, with the labor of
their hands alone, by their own measure of personal acuity.

Our Creator would not allow this faithlessness and perfidy to
continue, "So the Lord scattered them from there over all the earth,
and they stopped building the city. That is why it was called Babel.
The Lord confused the language of the whole world. From there the
Lord scattered them over the face of the whole earth" (Genesis 11:8-
9).

God's point of view. Humanity's point of view. Hypothesis. Proof.
Free will. Temptation. People needing to find out "why" for anything
and everything. The sciences and the humanities, philosophy and
theology thrive under the banner of "why" while searching for proof.

> *Why* is what drives not only everything we do, but
> also our emotional reactions to everything that
> happens to us. Imagine how quickly your frustration
> at encountering that traffic jam on your way home
> from work would turn into horror if, as you passed
> the accident that caused it, you caught a glimpse of
> a mangled corpse lying beside a totaled car. Or how
> easily the irritation you'd feel at being told you have
> to work an extra shift at work each week for the next
> two months might turn into a willingness to contribute
> when you learn the reason is that one of your
> colleagues was just diagnosed with cancer and needs to
> spend that time getting chemotherapy.

We're simply far more likely to accept a change if
we understand the reason for it. Interestingly, our
acceptance seems to hinge less on how much we like
the reason and more on how much sense the reason
makes to us. Even if the change fails to benefit us—
even if it causes us harm in some way—if our sense of
fairness is satisfied, we're far more likely to accept and
even embrace it. (https://www.psychologytoday.com/
us/blog/happiness-in-world/201011/why-we-need-
know-why)

So, why would God create the Tree of Knowledge in the first
place?

Why in the world would God create such a tree? If he
didn't want them to get tempted in the first place, he
should've removed all chances of temptation." But we
have to understand the necessity of the tree and why he
had to place it in the Garden.

God is a God of love. It comprises his entire being.
And if he wanted to give humans free will, something a
loving God would do, he had to allow for the possibility
for them to choose something over him, and therefore,
sin.

Think about it in this way. If someone creates a robot
and programs the machine to do a certain number of
functions, we wouldn't say the robot is capable of free
will or love. Free will and love come with a cost. We
learn the cost in Scripture. Because mankind chose to
use free will incorrectly, Jesus had to die on the cross.
(https://www.crosswalk.com/faith/bible-study/
what-sunday-school-didnt-teach-you-about-the-tree-
of-knowledge.html)

This sends shivers down my spine to think about it: Our Savior
died on a cross, made from the wood of a tree. A tree. Eating from

the forbidden tree of knowledge in the garden of Eden brought down mankind. *Wonder about that with me for a few minutes.*

Chapter Ten
Madness

Deception, Sorcery, Treachery

Personal point of view, free will, and temptation is a tricky mix.

Satan is called the Father of Lies for a reason. He capitalizes on man's search for knowledge and meaning for his benefit. He promises plenty and delivers hell.

He goes by many names: The Devil, Satan, Lucifer, the Prince of Darkness, the Father of Lies. Two of the biggest lies of the 21st century are that he doesn't exist and that hell isn't real.

He preys on man's search for meaning, plotting to destroy him. He tries to hijack God's holy order created in the frequencies and wavelengths of life, the rhythm of the ocean waves, the sounds of music, the vibrant colors of the world, a heartbeat, the very inhaling and exhaling of our breathing, relentlessly destroying, wreaking despair and destruction.

The enemy is a predator, scooping out remnants of joy and happiness from the hearts of men, slurping hopelessness in a gulp, wiping his face with man's tears. Feasting on the misery it causes, devouring mankind bit by bit, stealing children not yet born. He vomits misery and mayhem. He laughs at the madness he's left behind.

He taunts us, numbing us with alcohol, ruining us with drugs, all the while rendering us lukewarm, then cold-hearted, as our souls slip away. Reduced to a pile of rubbish, we no longer notice our stale breath, dead in the grief we can no longer feel. Care escapes us. Deep dread reigns in the enemy's nation.

> The Bible doesn't give us an exact timeline of Satan's origin. Rather, what we know of Satan's beginnings comes from passages written by the prophets Ezekiel and Isaiah, which passages Bible scholars believe detail the devil's fall from heaven (Ezekiel 28; Isaiah 14).
>
> The prophets tell us that Satan was an angel known as the "morning star," translated as Lucifer (Ezekiel

28:14; Isaiah 14:12). As an angel, Lucifer walked on God's holy mountain and was anointed to serve God as a member of the guardian cherubim, among the highest rank of angels in God's holy host second only to the seraphim (Ezekiel 28:14). That Lucifer was ordained a cherub was no small honor.

In heaven, the cherubim hold such a position of celestial prominence that God Himself sits "enthroned between the cherubim" (Isaiah 37:16).

As a creation of God, we know that Lucifer was created good (Genesis 1:31; Ezekiel 28:13). In fact, Scripture asserts that Lucifer started out as "blameless" in all his ways, and as the model of perfection, full of wisdom and perfect in beauty (Ezekiel 28:12-15). Further, God's ordination of Lucifer as a cherub demonstrates that God trusted Lucifer enough to give him a position of power among the heavenly angels (Ezekiel 28:14).

However, Lucifer wasn't satisfied with the power and gifts God gave him. Instead, Lucifer wanted more.

Lucifer became so consumed with pride over his God-given splendor that he became corrupt and violent, no longer willing to serve under God (Ezekiel 28:15-17; Isaiah 14:13-14). This sense of superiority led Lucifer to use his free will to scheme to be greater than God, and to assemble an army of angels to help him carry out that plot (Ezekiel 28:17; Isaiah 14:13-14; Revelation 12:3-4, Revelation 12:9).

Thus, Satan's sin was one of pride in rebelling against God and attempting to take from God the praise and glory reserved only for the Lord Almighty. Pride tops the list of sins that God hates (Proverbs 6:16-17). The pride that the Bible condemns doesn't refer to feelings of accomplishment over a job well done. Rather, pride in the Biblical sense refers to being so obsessed with yourself that your mind never turns to God and your heart never seeks Him (Psalm 10:4). Fortunately for us, Satan's prideful scheme to usurp God's throne failed.

As punishment for his disobedience and the grave dishonoring of his angelic post, God cast Lucifer out of heaven by hurling him and his army of fallen angels to Earth (Isaiah 14:15; Ezekiel 28:16-18; Revelation 12:9) and condemning them ultimately to hell (Matthew 25:41).

Jesus confirms the devil's fall from grace and likened it to lightning from heaven (Luke 10:18), and the Apostle Peter alluded to the devil's fall when he warned that God did not spare even the angels when they sinned but cast them into hell (2 Peter 2:4). Once Lucifer was thrown out of heaven, he realized that he didn't have the power to directly take God's throne from Him. Instead, Lucifer set his sights on overpowering God in another way—by tempting God's children to abandon Him. At this point, the "morning star" known as Lucifer became humankind's adversary and accuser, known as Satan.

Satan has been using his wisdom and wile to rob humanity of eternal salvation since his own fall from grace. In fact, Satan ushered in humanity's first sin by tempting Adam and Eve with much the same desire that caused his own fall—the sinful desire to be like God (Isaiah 14:13-14; Genesis 3:1-5).

Importantly, Satan's first temptation of mankind succeeded not only in straining humanity's relationship with God, but also in causing our first parents to turn against each other when Adam blamed Eve for giving him the forbidden fruit to eat (Genesis 3:12). This shows how easily temptation and sin can lead to conflict and division, furthering Satan's goal of creating chaos among God's children.

Compounding Satan's power is the fact that he isn't working alone. The army of angels that Satan assembled in his insurrection against God—one-third of the angels—now serve as demons doing Satan's bidding (Revelation 12:4-9). Demons are no less dangerous than Satan, as Scripture describes them as spiritual forces of evil (Ephesians 6:12) who can deceive, torment, and cause believers to do evil themselves (2 Corinthians 11:13-14; 2 Corinthians 12:7; Luke 22:3-4).

As believers, we know that Satan and his demons will ultimately be defeated and cast into the lake of fire for all eternity (Matthew 25:41). However, until the end times, Satan remains a powerful spiritual being whose sole aim is to deceive us into severing our relationship with God and with each other (John 8:44; Revelation 12:10).

It is by severing our relationship with God and with our brothers and sisters that Satan seeks to steal our peace and ultimately destroy our lives (John 10:10). It's no wonder that in describing the devil's attempts to unravel God's Kingdom, the Apostle Peter depicts Satan as a "roaring lion" that "prowls around...looking for someone to devour" (1 Peter 5:8). One way that the devil devours our relationship with God and with one another is by *tricking us into believing that what is right and wrong is relative.*

Satan wants nothing more than for each of us to act as our own individual gods, casting stones at each other based on our own moral code and denying the authority and commandments of the only God of the Universe. To avoid falling into Satan's traps, we need look no further than the cause of Satan's expulsion from paradise: pride. (https://www.crosswalk.com/faith/bible-study/why-was-satan-banished-in-the-bible.html)

Obviously, Satan completely hates God. While God is perfect and untouchable, Satan is aware that His children are neither. So, Satan goes after us, his mission is to push us to hurt one another and to turn our backs on our Creator.

> Scripture has quite a bit to say about Satan, yet most Christians are ignorant about him. God has written some adamant warnings about our enemy, and we need to heed them carefully. Many Christians are under constant attack by him but have no idea of the battle they're in. They think their lack of joy, broken relationships, and failures in life originate with them, when in reality their troubles are because they are following the voice of the enemy of their souls but are completely unaware of it.

> Satan is a liar and murderer. This part of him comes from his true nature, which, according to the Bible, consists of arrogance, vanity, envy, and selfish ambition. When we act in such a manner, we align ourselves with Satan as enemies of God. This is why the mark of a child of God is humility and absolute surrender to our Lord.

> Paul got to the essence of this idea in Philippians 2:3, where he wrote, "Do nothing out of rivalry or conceit, but in humility consider others as more important than yourselves." (https://promisekeepers.org/what-does-satan-want/)

Satan can't touch God, so, in his hatred and despair, he attacks God's children. He does it by appealing to the pride in each one of us. This enemy will use deception, sorcery, treachery, lies, anything it can use to separate us from the love of our Creator.

The enemy's motivation? Satan wants to steal God's children. After all, what is worse than losing a child you love? Satan can't create, so he kills.

How do we fight this misery? Where is God when we need Him? Let's explore what God has to say about all of this.

— End of Part One —

PART TWO

What Happened

Do not fear, for I have redeemed you;
I have called you by name; you are Mine!
Isaiah 43:1

85

Chapter Eleven

The Struggle Is Real

The Path to Holiness

Satan tricks and deceives, but Satan cannot create anything, nor can he take on human form. Many people think he can even though there is no Biblical basis for this misconception.

Satan is a created angel who was kicked out of Heaven. Most believe he was named Lucifer, who was kicked out because of pride (Ezek 28:12-19) and wanting to become like God (Isa 14:12-15). Based on (Rev 12:3-4,7-9), it appears that one-third of the other angels that God created fell with him. These are Satan's angels/demons. These created angels are spirit by nature (Heb 1:14) and invisible (2 Kin 6:16-17)(Num 22:22-31). God is also spirit (Jn 4:24), and invisible (Col 1:15)(1 Tim 1:17)(Heb 11:27). Jesus said that a spirit is not made up of flesh and bone (Lk 24:39)(Mt 16:17). God did give HIS angels human form in several places in the Bible (Heb 13:2)(Gen 18:1-16)(Lk 24:4), but nowhere is it shown in the Bible that angels/demons took on or can take on human form.

Having said this, it is important to understand that Satan and his angels/demons can clearly POSSESS people. This is shown in a number of places in the Bible (Lk 22:3)(Mk 7:25-30)(Lk 9:38-42). They can also possess animals (Mk 5:8-13)(Lk 8:32-33)(Mt 8:30-32), and I believe Satan possessed the snake in the Garden of Eden that tempted Eve into committing the first sin (Gen 3:1-15). Because neither Satan nor his angels/demons can take on human form, and do not have physical bodies, they can ONLY manipulate what God has already created, and cannot create something from nothing.

Satan can and does counterfeit many things that God
does, but he can only imitate, not create. (https://
jesusalive.cc/can-satan-create/)

Free will allows us to navigate our days without robotic
predetermination, we have been given the right to decide whether
or not to do this or that within the choices presented to us. We can
decide to make good, holy decisions or elect to make bad decisions
leading to perdition. It's up to us. God does not send anyone to
hell, grieving when his children turn away from Him. People send
themselves to hell. It's all in the decisions we make. We determine
our own outcome. James 4:7 tells us, "Submit therefore to God. But
resist the devil, and he will flee from you." We truly have no one to
blame but ourselves in the end.

We have to wonder if God ever regretted creating mankind, given
the constant caving to the enemy and the careless decisions we make
daily. Genesis 6:6 reveals, "So the Lord was sorry that He had made
mankind on the earth, and He was grieved in His heart."

So, did God regret creating us?

This is a reasonable question. Unlike most other
religions, in which God is presented as dispassionate,
the Bible presents God as possessing and being
influenced by powerful emotions. You can do your
own study (I am in London, in an airport, so will leave
the word studies to you), but the Bible presents God
as feeling love, anger, jealousy, compassion, mercy
and regret. It is possible to regret the result of one's
actions without feeling that the action was a mistake.
For example, if, in the process of designing a new
technology, someone might be killed when they use it.
One can regret the result, without feeling that the thing
was a mistake. I am sure that those who designed the
space shuttle program regretted that the Challenger
blew up, but still feel that developing the program
was, overall, a very good idea. We regret that allied

soldiers died in World War II, but we do not feel it was a mistake to fight the war. The alternative would have been worse.

I believe this applies to God's feeling of regret as expressed in Genesis. God created us because he wanted to love us, he wanted us to love him and he wanted us to love one another. Also, another purpose was so that we would glorify him. The result of God creating us was that all of these things did in fact happen. Nevertheless, this creation caused God great pain, as so many rebelled, and God felt regret.

I do not know if you are a parent, but I can tell you one thing for sure, which is that all parents have feelings of regret at times, and some more than others, especially when the child dies of disease at a very young age or has an extreme defect of some sort. Yet, these parents, despite their feelings of regret, do not feel that it was wrong to have a child. Like God, we all have mixed feelings.

I see Jesus in Matthew standing above Jerusalem, saying "O Jerusalem, Jerusalem." So many rejected him, but did he feel coming and dying for our sins was a mistake? Definitely not. In the same way, God does not feel that you and I are mistakes!!!! If you take the time, you can find literally hundreds of passages in the Bible in which God expresses his love for us and his satisfaction at those who love him.

So, the simple answer is this: No! God did not make a mistake when he created us with free will and with the ability to disobey him, but also to choose him and to love him. (https://evidenceforchristianity.org/if-god-regretted-making-human-beings-genesis-66-does-this-mean-that-god-made-a-mistake-what-does-this-say-about-god/)

God's Truth prevails. God's creation is flawless, including His gift of free will to us:

> The Nobel Prize winning physicist Sir William Bragg said, "Light brings us the news of the Universe." And the Bible agrees. Light does bring us the news, the good news, of the universe, directly from the Creator Himself. The message for us is crystal clear. Anyone who claims they can't see God and therefore can't believe in Him is being willfully blind. Romans 1:20 says it beautifully: "Since the creation of the world God's invisible qualities, His eternal power and divine nature, have been clearly seen, being understood from what has been made, so that people are without excuse." (Guillen, 2015, p. 82)

Viktor Frankel (1959), in his book *Mans Search for Meaning*, offers, "A human being is not one thing among others; things determine each other, but man is ultimately self-determining" (p. 133).

Indeed. We get to decide. Our Creator is generous. He is merciful. He loves us.

> Life and beauty and the capacity he gave us to enjoy them, all this God still gives and sustains, because he is still generous. As with each of his attributes, what God is, he is always and completely. God's generosity is enduring.
>
> We don't often hear about generosity when we study the attributes of God. But we do hear about his loving kindness and his goodness. His generosity is just the overflow of this love and goodness, motivating him to give.
>
> (https://www.ncfgiving.com/stories/the-generosity-of-god/)

"Your love, LORD, reaches to the heavens, your faithfulness to the skies. People take refuge in the shadow of your wings. They feast on the abundance of your house; you give them drink from your river of delights" (Psalm 36:5-8).

God beckons us to become holy with every breath we take. We do not understand His ways, though we do know what He commands of us, what He expects from us. God says, "This is My commandment, that you love one another, just as I have loved you" (John 15:12). Then, He makes it nearly impossible, "Therefore, you shall be perfect, as your heavenly Father is perfect" (Matthew 5:48).

I'll use myself as an example. I began smoking my junior year in college. At first, I used it as a prop on the stage of college life, journalism to be exact. A cigarette in hand, I instantly became an imaginary reporter in a dark and smoky room with a single light bulb suspended over my typewriter as I reported breaking news produced on the incoming newswires.

A friend was earning money part-time at a modeling studio downtown; I happily joined her. It didn't take long before I realized being a fashion model proved to be more interesting than sitting in a classroom. I squandered the tuition money my dad worked so hard to provide and began to party heartily.

I didn't finish school, breaking my father's heart. I continued to smoke for years. I knew I had to stop, but I couldn't. I was addicted. I smoked two packs a day for what seemed like forever.

Many years later, working as a closer at a title company, I was outside smoking during a work break. My co-workers had gone back to their desks; I lingered outside for a few more minutes, deciding to light up one more before going inside. I inhaled deeply. I knew I had to quit. I prayed to quit. Then, something strange happened.

I looked up and saw a nicely-dressed gentleman standing about an-arm-and-a-half's length in front of me. I was startled because I had been deep in thought and didn't see him approaching. I vividly recall he had very kind eyes which softened the startle. He smiled and said, "I overheard you telling your co-workers you needed to stop smoking." He continued, "I went through that a few years ago and haven't smoked since."

I politely asked him to tell me how he had been able to stop smoking. He answered, "Pray often. Pray a lot."

I told him I prayed a lot already and thanked him for his advice. I reached for the door to go back inside, not wanting to continue this conversation with a stranger. As I opened the door, he said this, "Ask God to smoke for you."

This, of course, stopped me dead in my tracks. *What a strange thing to say*, I thought.

The stranger continued talking to me, adding, "*God loves you and doesn't want you to be sick. Smoking won't make Him sick, let Him smoke for you. Every time you want a cigarette, ask Him to smoke it for you.*"

There was a sense of urgency in his voice.

It seemed as though time stopped. I really don't know how long I stood there, but when I looked up, he was gone. I searched the area with my eyes and there was not a sign of him anywhere.

There is absolutely no way I could have thought this up on my own. I had to admit that it did make sense, though. God could not get sick. He could take my addiction from me. God could relieve me, prevent me from getting sick, all I had to do was *ask Him to smoke for me.* A strange feeling of protection, care and calmness, of love, swept over me as I opened the door and headed back to my work area.

I didn't say anything when I returned to my desk because the whole thing seemed too big and too outlandish to tell anyone at work. I felt the need to sort it all out, and think, and sort some more.

A few days later, on April 23rd, 2004, at 5:04 CDT (I glanced at my watch), I inhaled, exhaled, and tossed my last cig out the window of my car. I looked in the rearview mirror and watched it bounce on the pavement. Yes, I littered in the throes of a Miracle.

It has been said that God chooses the biggest sinners and uses them to show His mercy and love. I have to agree, because in the following days He must have smoked a few hundred cigarettes for me.

The cravings became less and less as the days passed. It was totally amazing. I would think about having a cigarette (every few minutes at first) and as soon as I asked Him to smoke it for me, the thought immediately was gone until the next time I wanted one. The times got further and further apart until I really didn't think about smoking at all anymore.

"That was almost twenty years ago. I truly do believe God sent a messenger to me that day at work. Thank you, dear Lord Jesus." (Krueger & Nelson, 2017, p. 117)

I knew I had broken my father's heart over and over, and apologized many times to him. He loved me. He forgave me. I knew I had broken God's heart over and over many times. He continued to love me. I asked for forgiveness, He forgave me. I changed my ways. I repented. He healed me of my addiction.

God knows we fail to make good decisions, and we make ourselves sick. He heals us in His time, His way, when we turn to Him. My Dad knew this about our Creator and made sure I knew it, too.

God alone can make us holy, and that happens when we go to Him and let Him. Sometimes, He sends people to each one of us so we can show His love to them too, until they can see it for themselves.

As our loving Father instructs us all, "As obedient children, do not be conformed to the former lusts which were yours in your ignorance, but like the Holy One who called you, be holy yourselves also in all your behavior; because it is written: 'You shall be holy, for I am holy.'" (1 Peter 1:14-16).

God's love and protection, like a good Father's, is forever.

Chapter Twelve

God's Protection Is Forever

Temptation Is Everywhere

God allows us to decide our own fate, while specifically warning us to not participate in the evil activities of sorcerers, magicians, and liars. Deuteronomy 18:10-12 instructs us not to participate in any form of witchcraft, magic, divination, and not to contact mediums because it is detestable to Him. God is explicit in His command to us to not participate in witchcraft, nor are we to seek out magic. God knows these detestable actions will turn into addictions, ruining us.

Addiction, whether to cigarettes, drugs, sex, or the occult, is slavery to sin and direct rebellion against God. Addiction represents the worldly way of seeking comfort and relief apart from God, when our Creator is our only real source of hope and help (Philippians 3:18-19).

God's Word distinctly warned the Israelites in Leviticus 19:31, "Do not turn to mediums or seek out spiritists, for you will be defiled by them. I am the Lord your God." Magic is directly related to demons through the practice of the occult, often referred to as the dark arts.

Demons are fallen angels who joined Satan in his rebellion against God. They were defeated and cast out of heaven along with Satan (Revelation 12:7-9). Demons continue to serve Satan in his quest to tempt mankind to turn their backs on God, too.

Psalm 18:30 reminds us, "As for God, His way is blameless; The word of the LORD is refined; He is a shield to all who take refuge in Him. The Psalmist tells us, "As for God, His way is perfect."

Since God's ways are without error, we can trust that whatever He does, whatever He allows, is perfect. Isaiah 55:8-9 reminds us, "For My thoughts are not your thoughts, nor are your ways My ways," declares the LORD. "For as the heavens are higher than the earth, So are My ways higher than your ways, and My thoughts than your thoughts."

Satan tempted the ancient Egyptians to practice magic during the time of Moses and Joseph. The Pharaoh's sorcerers were busy trying to duplicate the miracles God was working through Moses and Aaron (Exodus 7 & Exodus 8). Within the Book of Exodus, God condemns to death anyone who participates in sorcery or magic.

Ancient rulers were condemned for evil practices, including sorcery in 2 Chronicles 33:6,

> And he burned his sons as an offering in the Valley of the Son of Hinnom, and used fortune-telling and omens and sorcery, and dealt with mediums and with necromancers. He did much evil in the sight of the LORD, provoking him to anger.

Sorcerers were prevalent in ancient Egypt (Exodus 7:11; Isaiah 19:3), and the kingdom of Babylon, with King Nebuchadnezzar (Jeremiah 27:9; Daniel 2:2). The Prophet Malachi also tells of God's judgment on those involved in sorcery: "Then I will draw near to you for judgment. I will be a swift witness against the sorcerers" (Malachi 3:5).

The use of spells, divination, or speaking to spirits, is fully condemned in the Bible. The word "sorcery" describes an evil or deceptive practice. Sorcery attempts to bypass God's power and wisdom in an effort to give acclaim and praise to Satan instead.

The word "sorcery" is derived from the Greek word *pharmakeia*, which translates to the word *pharmacy* in the English language. In early New Testament days, the word *pharmakeia* essentially meant "dealing in poison" or "drug use," and was applied to the use of divination and spell casting. "Biblical 'sorcery' seems to be about abusing drugs for idolatry, recreation, and/or oppression of others." (https://www.gotquestions.org/pharmakeia-in-the-Bible.html)

Sorcerers often used illicit drugs along with their incantations and amulets to conjure occult power from Satan.

Today's use of the word *sorcery* brings to mind images of supernatural power and spells, while the biblical use of the word *pharmakeia* suggests various forms of drug abuse as is used in pagan worship, or a drug addiction, or as a poison used to manipulate and control others.

Bernie Shrine, a professional magician writes,

> I have been a life-long magician, both as a performer
> and creator of magical effects. This art of manipulation,
> misdirection, and deception has taught me a sobering
> life lesson to be careful what you choose to believe.
> There is a thin line between reality and illusion, and
> every great trick has a flaw. The magician's task is to
> minimize, disguise, or justify the flaw. Be assured that
> every time a mind-reader puts on a blindfold, it is so
> the mentalist can see and the audience can't determine
> where he is looking. The very tool that is supposed to
> prevent trickery enables it.
>
> (https://www.huffpost.com/entry/the-art-of-
> deception-a-ma_b_8161274)

Isaiah 44:20 reminds us, "He feeds on ashes; a deceived heart has misled him. And he cannot save himself, nor say, 'Is there not a lie in my right hand,'" We remember, "The heart is more deceitful than all else and is desperately sick; Who can understand it?" Jeremiah 17:9.

Old Testament Prophet Obadiah tells us, "The arrogance of your heart has deceived you, The one who lives in the clefts of the rock, On the height of his dwelling place, Who says in his heart, 'Who will bring me down to earth'" (Obadiah 1:3).

Pride promises exaltation, while delivering shame and condemnation instead.

Sorcery is "the use of power gained from the assistance or control of evil spirits especially for divining." (https://www.merriam-webster.com/dictionary/sorcery)

"Pride goes before destruction, And a haughty spirit before stumbling" (Proverbs 16:18). Satan knows this and uses anything he can to his advantage to steal your soul from our Creator. He, and his demonic minions, use sorcery, drugs, and magic, to tempt us in an effort to lure us into hell with him. Satan hates God. Stealing God's children is his hateful act of revenge against Him.

God knows this, reminding us over and over of His love for us, how He is always there for us.

Chapter Thirteen

Forgiveness, Mercy, and Direction

God Is With Us in Our Suffering

Satan tempts us; we capitulate, stumbling over our own pride of self, thinking we know what is better for us than the One who created us. Messes are caused by our own bad decisions. We suffer. We succumb to sin; we suffer more. We become serfs of Satan; we suffer at the hands of those who have already given their souls to the enemy. No one is exempt from temptation. The deceiver beckons us with promises of earthly comforts, fame and glory, we are allowed to make a deadly decision, subsequently falling into the pits of despair with him.

> Demon spirits can invade and indwell human bodies. It is their objective to do so. By indwelling a person they obtain greater advantage in controlling that person than when they are working from the outside. When demons indwell a person, he or she is said to "have" evil spirits, to be "with" evil spirits, or to be "possessed" with demons. The word "possessed" by the King James version is the Greek word *daimonizomai*. Many Greek authorities say this is not an accurate translation. It should be translated as "demonized" or "have demons." Much misunderstanding has resulted from the word "possessed." This word suggests total ownership. In this sense, a Christian could never be "demon possessed." He could not be owned by demons because he is owned by Christ. (Hammond, 1973, p. 9)

Let's look at this another way:

> There was no lack in Adam and Eve's lives; they had every reason to be perfectly content. Yet when the serpent suggested to Eve that there was something she didn't have, something she really needed to be happy, namely, the wisdom that would come from eating from the forbidden tree of knowledge and the taste

experience of eating its delicious fruit, Eve allowed the perspective of the serpent to shape her perspective. Rather than being content with all the goodness showered in her and surrounding her, Eve began to see an empty place in her life, in her diet, in her knowledge, in her experience. Her desire for something more, something other than God's provision, combined with her growing doubts about God's goodness, led her to reach out for what she thought would make her happy, fulfilled, and satisfied.

The very thing that was supposed to bring joy and satisfaction now would bring pain and frustration. (Guthrie, 2018, p.18)

Sin disconnects us from God, "But your iniquities have separated you from your God; And your sins have hidden His face from you, so that He will not hear" (Isaiah 59:2). Suffering moves us to search for God, to seek His Holy Face, to trust Him.

Deeply desperate, David, the shepherd in the Old Testament, cries out to God, "How long, O Lord? Will You forget me forever? How long will You hide Your face from me" (Psalm 13:1)

God teaches us patience, while confirming His faithfulness. We realize we have been being guided all along by the loving hand of our Creator. His hand sturdily on our backs, we trudge up that steep hill toward Him, away from our sinful selves; we finally understand His forgiveness and mercy. We rejoice at the opportunity to tell others of His love. He allows us to see a glimpse of His Greatness, He lets us feel His forever love for us. We come to the place where we are no longer ashamed, we are forgiven.

Then, we see the tears of the innocent, those who have not offended God and are suffering. Job's story, in the Old Testament, tells the story of a righteous man whom God allowed the devil to test. Job's life fell away bit by bit until he was sitting on the ground covered with boils, his family dead, his business wrecked, and with real morons for friends.

Regrettably, Job's friends are not able to endure the mystery of his suffering, so they jump to conclusions about its source. The first of the three, Eliphaz, acknowledges that Job has been a source of strength to others (Job 4:3-4). But then he turns and puts the blame for Job's suffering squarely on Job himself. "Think now," he says, "who that was innocent ever perished? Or where were the upright cut off? As I have seen, those who plow iniquity and sow trouble reap the same" (Job 4:7-8). Job's second friend, Bildad, says much the same. "See, God will not reject a blameless person nor take the hand of evildoers" (Job 8:20). The third friend, Zophar, repeats the refrain. "If iniquity is in your hand, put it far away, do not let wickedness reside in your tents. Surely then you will lift up your face without blemish; you will be secure, and will not fear....Your life will be brighter than the noonday" (Job 11:14-15, 17).

(https://www.theologyofwork.org/old-testament/job/jobs-friends-blame-job-for-the-calamity-job-4-23/jobs-friends-accuse-him-of-doing-evil-job-4-23)

In other words, "Oh, you must have done something terrible to deserve this Job," his friends seemed to say. Yet, Job hadn't done anything to deserve it. He was innocent.

Ultimately the only answer God gave to Job was a revelation of Himself. It was as if God said to him, "Job, I am your answer." Job was not asked to trust a plan but a person, a personal God who is sovereign, wise, and good. It was as if God said to Job: "Learn who I am. When you know me, you know enough to handle anything. (Sproul, 2010, p. 141)

Chad Bird (2019), author and lecturer, tells us of God's divine pursuit of His children in Psalm 23:

In verse 6, we read, "Surely goodness and mercy shall follow me all the days of my life." The verb for "follow" is *radaph*. But the translation of this Hebrew verb as "follow" is far too weak and bloodless.

Radaph means to chase after, to pursue. The goodness and mercy of God do not follow us like a good little puppy dog, trailing along behind us. Rather, they gallop after us like a celestial stallion. As in the famous poem by Francis Thompson, the Lord's goodness and mercy chase us down labyrinthine paths like the Hound of Heaven. They stay hot on our heels. The divine love and grace of our shepherd *radaph* us all the way to heaven's gate and into the arms of our waiting Father. We are pursued by mercy. We are chased by grace. We are not merely followed. (https://www.1517.org/articles/three-hidden-hebrew-treasures-in-psalm-23)

There is pain and misery we cannot see at all with our earthly eyes. So often, this silent prayer is whispered, almost in secret between us and our Creator, "Do you even hear me, Lord? I am miserable."

The suffering that began in the garden of Eden is evident throughout the Old Testament. The prophet Micaiah suffered deeply. He was repeatedly slapped in the face, insulted, and sent to prison for telling the truth (1 Kings 22:24-28). The prophet Jeremiah was beaten and put in prison (Jeremiah 37:14-21). The prophets Amos (1 Kings 7:10-12), and Uriah (Jeremiah 26:20-23) all suffered persecution. Why? Because they preached the will of God during politically adverse circumstances of their time. They trusted God; they knew His Truth.

God knows that when times are difficult, we may doubt His presence with us and His mercy toward us. The actions of the Israelites after God mercifully delivered them in Egypt, where they were subjected to slavery for centuries, exemplifies this perfectly:

- When the Egyptian army bore down on them at the Red Sea, the Israelites believed that they would die there.

- When their food began to run out in the wilderness, the Israelites believed that they would starve.

- When their camp had no water, the Israelites believed that they would die of thirst.

- When they got tired of eating only manna, the Israelites believed that God really didn't care about them.

- When Moses was on Mt. Sinai for 40 days, the Israelites made a golden calf to worship.

Even when the Israelites doubted, God came through for them. So why did they doubt God, again and again? Why do we? It's because, in the stress of the moment, we forget how God has helped us in the past, and we forget God's promises, which He always keeps. We need to trust in God. After all, His way is perfect, His Word is flawless, and, if we take refuge in him, then He will shield us. Every time.

(https://www.crosswalk.com/faith/bible-study/4-things-the-old-testament-teaches-about-suffering.html)

Satan, the ultimate trickster, will continue to spin his web of deceit, setting a trap of misery for us to fall into if we are not sober and alert to his ways. If we are not paying attention, focused on the love of our Creator, we will trip time and time again over our own pride. We will mistakenly think we will be better off, only to end up wallowing in the misery of our mistake.

We need God's help to get through this world ruled by the enemy.

Chapter Fourteen
A World Needing Help

Magic and Misery

For the teraphim speak iniquity,
And the diviners see lying visions
And tell false dreams;
They comfort in vain.
Therefore the people wander like sheep,
They are afflicted, because there is no shepherd.

Zechariah 10:2

Written around 500 years before the birth of Jesus Christ, the Prophet Zechariah foretold with uncanny accuracy of the coming of a Messiah who would save humanity from its repeated transgressions, from its willful debauchery.

> But Zechariah didn't stop there. He went into great detail about Christ's Second Coming, providing a treasure trove of information about the End Times. The book is often difficult to understand, packed with symbolism and vivid imagery, yet its predictions about a future Savior jump out with crystal clarity.
>
> (https://www.learnreligions.com/book-of-zechariah-4036303)

The days were filled with treacherous examples of mankind's disobedience:

> There are numerous references to sorcery, witchcraft, magic, divination, omen interpretation, astrology, and other dark arts throughout the Bible. In Deut. 18:10-11, the Lord commands, "Let no one be found among you who sacrifices his son or daughter in the fire, who practices divination or sorcery, interprets omens, engages in witchcraft, or casts spells, or who is a medium or spiritist or who consults the dead (NIV)." In 2 Kings 9:22, we read that Jezebel practiced witchcraft. Jewish and Israelite kings practiced magic, sorcery, witchcraft, and others, most notably the very evil Manasseh (2 Chron. 33:6) and his son Amon (verse 22).
>
> (https://believersweb.org/the-truth-about-magic-witchcraft-and-sorcery/)

What did King Manasseh do that the Bible described as evil? Reigning about 600 years before the birth of Christ, he was the son of the beloved, good King Hezekiah. Manasseh reversed the acts of his father, committing atrocities against the people of Judah who were not loyal to him.

Manasseh built shrines to idols, and restored the polytheistic worship of Baal and Asherah (2 Kings 21) in Solomon's Temple in Jerusalem. He implemented the Assyrian astral cult, the worship of the stars, the planets, and other heavenly bodies as deities, throughout Judah.

King Manasseh was passionate in his worship of false gods, reportedly participating in the sacrificial cult of Moloch, a bull-headed idol with outstretched hands over a fire, which consisted of sacrificing young children by passing them through fire (2 Kings 21:6).

2 Kings 21:10 suggests that several prophets warned the people of Judah to not participate in the rituals promoted by Manasseh. Manasseh's response was to persecute those who disagreed with him. The opposing prophets were slaughtered (Jeremiah 2:30). Innocent blood was shed on the streets of Jerusalem, and for many decades those who sympathized with prophetic ideas were in constant danger.

It's important to note here:

> All the immoral, the ethical, the religious, the self-righteous, the atheist, the agnostic, the king, the commoner . . . the young and the old are caught within the Scripture's web of confinement due to sin. "Man" in the Greek Scriptures is *huph hamartian*, man under sin. This means he is under the power of, in subjection to, under the control of or dependent upon, sin. Sin holds man under its authority, just as a child is under his parents or an army is under its commander. It is viewed as a living, active, forceful and dynamic power that has man under its sway.

(https://www.cgg.org/index.cfm/library/article/
id/489/what-sin-is-does.htm)

Recall where it all started:

> The ten commandments were first made known to
> Adam in the Garden of Eden. Why? Because that is the
> very law that he broke in the "original" sin. EVERY
> ONE of the ten commandments was then in full force
> and effect. It was SIN to transgress any one of them
> between the time of Adam and Moses. You can read
> this in your own Bible.

> Every one of the ten commandments WAS IN
> EXISTENCE during the time of Adam. It was SIN to
> break any one of them PRIOR to the time of the law
> of Moses. The law of Moses, we know, didn't come
> UNTIL the time of Moses—430 years after the time
> of Abraham. But the SPIRITUAL LAW has been in
> existence from Adam!

> The original sin is recorded in Genesis, beginning with
> chapter 2, verse 15: "And the Eternal took the man and
> put him in the garden of Eden to dress it and keep it.
> And the Eternal God commanded the man saying, "Of
> every tree of the garden thou mayest freely eat."

> God gave him permission. God is Supreme Ruler.
> God is giving the orders. He is teaching. The man
> DIDN'T KNOW. The man had to be TOLD. He
> had to be TAUGHT and INSTRUCTED. Here is the
> instruction—the command, and a sentence. Notice:
> "But of the tree of the knowledge of good and evil,"
> a MIXTURE of good and evil, "of the tree of the
> knowledge of good and evil, thou shalt not eat of it; for
> in the day that thou eatest thereof, thou shalt SURELY
> DIE!"

"The wages of sin is death." God was preaching the gospel of the man. There it is! The very fact that God said, "In the day that thou eatest thereof ..." shows that the man was ALLOWED to do it, that the man was a FREE MORAL AGENT, that the man himself had to make the choice. God designed that you and I CHOOSE whether or not we will obey His law, or not.

Animals don't make a choice. Animals have instinct.

God ordained that you and I must make a choice. And if we choose the right way to live, according to that law which God set in motion to produce happiness and contentment and a FULL, THRIVING, ENJOYABLE life, we can have it. But if we're going to choose to live the other way, we're going to have suffering, sorrows and curses—that's what we've elected to do. (https://www.cgg.org/index.cfm/library/booklet/id/744/were-ten-commandments-before-moses.htm)

The gift of free will in mankind, proved to be heartbreaking over and over to our Creator God. Yes, there were good men and women, doing their utmost to serve their Lord God. Yet, there were those who succumbed to the wiles of Satan, wreaking havoc on those who were doing their best to obey God and to honor His gift of life to them.

Victor Frankl (1959), reminds us in *Man's Search for Meaning*:

"What matters, therefore, is not the meaning of life in general but rather the specific meaning of a person's life at a given moment ... to put the question in general terms would be comparable to the question posed to a chess champion: "Tell me, Master, what is the best move in the world?" There simply is no such thing as the best or even a good move apart from a particular situation in a game and the particular personality of one's opponent." (p. 108)

Our opponent, the serpent, the magician, the deceiver, is Satan himself. He slithers into our lives when we least expect him, our guard down, knowing full well our next move could prove to be deadly. Satan is capable of corrupting entire civilizations, one person at a time.

A wise, beloved professor was asked this question: "If our God is a loving and just, merciful God, how could He kill the people in an entire country, how could He annihilate entire civilizations, flood His entire world saving only a few people?" His answer, in the form of two questions, was brilliant in its graceful simplicity, "Why would our Creator, who had given us everything we need to survive and thrive, keep people around who will never love Him, who will never worship Him? And, why would He keep people around who hurt His beloved children?"

Our Creator is a loving God who covers us with His protection. Psalm 91:4 reminds us, "He will cover you with His pinions, and under His wings you may take refuge; His faithfulness is a shield and wall."

The magician is no match.

Our Creator loves us so much, He decided to rescue us from the oppression of the serpent and those who worship the serpent, by sending a Savior.

Chapter Fifteen

God Sends a Savior

Love

Before proceeding to the event that changed the course of the world's history, including the number of the year itself, let's look at the timeline of events:

The Bible gives us dates to work with starting in Genesis chapters 5 & 11. "Adam lived one hundred and thirty years, and begat a son in his own likeness, after his image; and called his name Seth" (Genesis 5:3). Chapter 5 ends with Noah who, at five hundred years of age, "begat Shem, Ham and Japheth." You will notice that these ages are "round numbers," that is between Adam and Seth, there could have been 130 years, and 2 months, 3 days, etc. So, is the Bible recording it as exactly 130 years means it could have been even 131 years or 128 years, rounded to 130 years. The Bible does not give us any more detail re: these numbers, but using the laws of math, 130 years could mean anywhere from 126 to 134 years, rounded to 130 years. At least that was what I was taught in math class.

But throwing in Genesis 11, you get the "round" number of 1656 years from Adam to the birth of Abram (Abraham). Further studies of ancient records place Abraham around 2100 to 2000 BC and Moses about 1440 BC, David 1000 BC, etc. Note that the Septuagint (a Greek translation of the Old Testament done about 300 BC) adds several hundred years (1300 years to be exact) to the record, and we just do not know whether that was mistranslation or a deliberate attempt to falsify the ancient Hebrew text. Suffice it to say that through ancient records and the Bible text alone, you come to about 4000 years between Adam's creation and the birth of Christ. Since we now stand

at 2016 AD, Bible records indicate a total of roughly
6000 years from creation to the present.

(https://www.blogos.org/exploringtheword/adam-
Jesus-timeline.php)

And for anyone who has swallowed a piece of fruit from the tree
called Darwinism,

> Darwinian evolutionists of course, decry such a young
> creation and claim billions of years from the creation
> of the universe to the present; obviously either the
> Bible records are faulty or the theory of evolution is
> simply false. Some Christians try to force in additional
> time with various schemes, theories to reconcile the
> "science so-called" that is evolution, and a "big bang"
> with the Bible. There are many reasons why those
> attempts fail. There was no death until Adam's sin
> about 6000 years ago, so how then do we account for
> the fossil record, little local floods over millions and
> billions of years, or one global flood as described in the
> Bible about 4500 years ago?! Peter tells us "whereby
> the world that then was, being overflowed with water,
> perished" (2 Peter 3:6). Peter is of course speaking of
> the global flood in the days of Noah.

> One needs to only examine historical records to know
> that we have pretty complete records for civilizations
> that existed down to the village and town (tribe) level
> up to 6 or 7 thousand years ago, and none earlier
> than that. Who wrote the history of 120,000 BC for
> example? Obviously, no one. Yet according to one
> scheme of man's history, hominids no different than
> modern man existed up to 2 or 3 million years ago,
> and these "men and women" not physically different
> from us were not able to start recording history until 6
> thousand years ago. Or could it be that history started
> 6 thousand years ago because that is when God created

the universe and Adam and Eve? I leave that to your scholarship and wisdom to decide. Since Adam was created "very good," I doubt he lacked intelligence or ingenuity, and he lived much longer than any of us do today; so, he had plenty of time to figure out a written code. Even the native American Indians, who supposedly did not write, used colored beads (wampum) to record their histories, a method of code no longer available today, long lost.

(https://www.blogos.org/exploringtheword/adam-Jesus-timeline.php)

Throughout the history of His magnificent creation, God has provided for us a roadmap, complete with specific directions. God spoke of signs and specific circumstances through His prophets. These prophets predicted the events mankind should watch for, so the Savior would be recognized and believed when He arrived on earth.

These signs or prophecies were given to us in the Old Testament. The Old Testament is the part of the Bible written before Jesus was born. Its writings were completed in 450 B.C. The Old Testament, written hundreds of years before Jesus' birth, contains over 300 prophecies that Jesus fulfilled through His life, death and resurrection.

Mathematically speaking, the odds of anyone fulfilling this amount of prophecy are staggering. Mathematicians put it this way:

1 person fulfilling 8 prophecies: 1 in 100,000,000,000,000,000 1 person fulfilling 48 prophecies: 1 chance in 10 to the 157th power 1 person fulfilling 300+ prophecies: Only Jesus!

It is the magnificent detail of these prophecies that mark the Bible as the inspired Word of God. Only God could foreknow and accomplish all that was written about Christ. This historical accuracy and reliability sets the Bible apart from any other book or record.

(https://www1.cbn.com/biblestudy/biblical-prophecies-fulfilled-by-jesus)

The times were turbulent when our Savior came into this world. The Roman general Pompey had conquered Jerusalem and the adjacent areas around 63 BC. The Romans deposed the ruling Hasmonean dynasty of Judaea which had been in power since 140 BC. Then, the Roman Senate declared Herod the Great "King of the Jews " circa 40 BC. Subsequently, Judea proper, including Samaria and Idumea became the Roman province of Judaea in 6 CE.

God's chosen people in Israel were under the oppressive rule of Rome. There were Roman guards, called to police the city of David, Jerusalem. Although no longer slaves living in a foreign land, they had returned only to become exiles in their own country. Their own temple was built by an outsider, Herod the Great, who was from a rival nation. Political oppression reigned.

The nation of Israel was falling apart. Four groups in Israel were fighting against each other, each one trying to become the leader of the people. Residing in Jerusalem, the legalistic Pharisees attempted to shape religious life in Israel with their elaborate traditions. There were the Sadducees, who opposed the legalism of the Pharisees, choosing to embrace the Law of Moses. Holding an influential place in the temple, they were considered to be the lawyers at the time. They were in charge of the courts of law.

Meanwhile, the Essenes, who lived near Qumran in a commune of sorts, were the scribes preserving the Dead Sea Scrolls. They lived simple, uncomplicated lives in seclusion. Completely devoted to God, they prayed, begging Him to send a good leader to overthrow Rome.

Finally, the Zealots were an overly enthusiastic group of men who did not pray for change, deciding they would rather take matters into their own hands. They engaged in violent means to overthrow

Roman rule. "The result of these four competing sects in Judaism led to constant friction, only increased by the oppressive rule of Rome. Riots were common. Tension was unceasing. Darkness permeated Judaism." (https://davidschrock.com/2011/12/12/darkness-the-world-in-which-christ-was-born/)

The Jewish people were embittered by Roman rule, preferring to self-rule. They deeply resented the fact that the Roman administrators could appoint the Jewish High Priest and remove him from office on a whim. The Jewish people begged God to send them a savior, a strong leader who would free them from the tyranny of Roman rule.

Then, it happened ...

The Savior was born.

They were expecting a King. They wanted a Warrior.

The last thing they expected was a baby in a smelly stable in a manger.

Our Creator would have it no other way.

Our Savior grew up.

He showed us how to love. He taught us how to forgive.

And then, despite all of the Miracles, the healings, the pomp and the glory,

they killed Him.

There were only two people with Him when He died.

His Mom and His best friend, John.

The Savior tore the veil separating earth from heaven.

He crushed the serpent.

They thought He was dead forever. They thought it was the end.

The impossible became possible.

He rose from death, alive again, conquering the enemy.

Then, they watched Him leave earth, they watched Him go up,

ascending into the heavens.

They were so scared without Him. They didn't want to be tortured and

persecuted like He was.

They were ashamed of themselves for being such cowards.

They locked themselves into an upstairs room,

far away from the madding crowd.

And then it happened.

Again.

He sent His Holy Spirit to comfort them and to give them strength.

Just like He said He would.

His name was Jesus. He conquered death.

His Holy Spirit is with us to this day.

Chapter Sixteen

Jesus Sends Us a Helper

Equipped and Ready

God had sent this world our Savior, conquering the serpent and all demons, promising eternal life to earth's citizens, to each one of His beloved children. Witnesses to Jesus' death and resurrection were commissioned by our Savior Himself to tell people about what had happened.

> And Jesus came up and spoke to them, saying, "All authority in heaven and on earth has been given to Me. Go, therefore, and make disciples of all the nations, baptizing them in the name of the Father and the Son and the Holy Spirit, teaching them to follow all that I commanded you; and behold, I am with you always, to the end of the age" (Matthew 28:18-20).

> So, when they had come together, they began asking Him, saying, "Lord, is it at this time that You are restoring the kingdom to Israel?" But He said to them, "It is not for you to know periods of time or appointed times which the Father has set by His own authority; but you will receive power when the Holy Spirit has come upon you; and you shall be My witnesses both in Jerusalem and in all Judea, and Samaria, and as far as the remotest part of the earth" (Acts 1:6-8).

Within days after His Holy Resurrection, Jesus ascended into the heavens, promising to send his disciples a "Comforter and Helper." Jesus said,

> "I will ask the Father, and He will give you another Helper, so that He may be with you forever; the Helper is the Spirit of truth, whom the world cannot receive, because it does not see Him or know Him; but you know Him because He remains with you and will be in you" (John 14:16-17).

Although Jesus' personal ministry on earth had ended, His glorious act of Redemption brought forth His new ministry of love and mercy on earth in His new church.

Jesus' disciples didn't understand that, yet. When Jesus' disciples, friends, and followers were gathered together in that upper room in Jerusalem nine days after His ascension into the heavens, they were huddled together in fear, trying to avoid persecution for their new beliefs.

Praying together for safety, protection and direction, this gathering could be considered to be the first church service in His new church, the Body of Christ, after Jesus' ascension into heaven. This gathering together was in obedience to Jesus' final instructions to His disciples,

> He commanded them not to leave Jerusalem, but to
> wait for what the Father had promised, "Which," He
> said, "you heard of from Me; for John baptized with
> water, but you will be baptized with the Holy Spirit not
> many days from now" (Acts 1:4-5).

This first meeting of believers occurred on one of the Jewish feast days known as the Feast of Harvest or the Feast of Weeks, thereafter known as Pentecost. This particular day is mentioned in five places in the first five books of the Bible: Exodus 23, Exodus 24, Leviticus 16, Numbers 28, and Deuteronomy 16.

It was in this upper room that His Holy Spirit descended upon them, just as Jesus had told them He would:

> "I will not leave you as orphans; I am coming to you.
> After a little while, the world no longer is going to see
> Me, but you are going to see Me; because I live, you
> also will live. On that day you will know that I am in My
> Father, and you are in Me, and I in you. The one who
> has My commandments and keeps them is the one who
> loves Me; and the one who loves Me will be loved by
> My Father, and I will love him and will reveal Myself to
> him" (John 14:18-21).

Great joy and an abundance of spiritual strength was found in Jesus' followers after receiving the gift of the Holy Spirit. They understood Jesus' words as to why He had to leave the earth and what He meant when we said He would send them a Helper, a Comforter.

Two remarkable things happened to the disciples after receiving the gift of the Holy Spirit on Pentecost:

> The first is that they "returned to Jerusalem with great joy" (Luke 24:52). They were not despondent over the departure of Jesus. Obviously, they finally understood why He was leaving. They understood what, for the most part, the church since then has failed to understand. We live as if it would not have been better for Jesus to leave.
>
> The second obvious change in the lives of the disciples was in their spiritual strength. After Pentecost, they were different people. No longer did they flee like sheep without a shepherd. Instead, they turned the world upside down. They turned the world upside down because they fully understood two simple things: the "where" and the "why" of Jesus' departure. (https://www.christianity.com/jesus/early-church-history/pentecost/what-changes-happened-after-penecost.html)

Filled with His Holy Spirit, they went forth from that first gathering, that first church service, filled with love, strength and the gifts of the Holy Spirit. They were equipped to take on the destructive forces of the enemy. With these gifts, they were ready and equipped to minister to God's people:

> But to each one is given the manifestation of the Spirit for the common good. For to one is given the word of wisdom through the Spirit, and to another the word of knowledge according to the same Spirit; to another faith by the same Spirit, and to another gifts of healing by the one Spirit, and to another the effecting of

miracles, and to another prophecy, and to another the distinguishing of spirits, to another various kinds of tongues, and to another the interpretation of tongues. But one and the same Spirit works all these things, distributing to each one individually just as He wills (1 Corinthians 12:7-11).

Our Creator knew His followers, those who loved Him, needed help. The enemy was furious.

Chapter Seventeen:

The Father of Lies Is Furious

Sorcerers and Thieves

Satan was enraged. He knew had to sharpen his skills and come up with sneakier ways to deceive God's children. He had to devise plans to "recreate" God's perfect creation. Furious because he could not and would never be able to create life, he set out to corrupt God's magnificent creation.

Satan uses magic to skew reality in order to confuse and manipulate.

This is an old trick of the enemy, used from the beginning of God's creation. The prophet Ezekiel boldly tells of the depth and extent of magic. Ezekiel tells us that magic spells are real and are used as snares to trap God's people in order to control their destinies by usurping their faith.

Ezekiel offers this,

> Therefore, this is what the Lord GOD says: "Behold, I am against your magic bands by which you capture souls there as birds, and I will tear them from your arms; and I will let them go, those souls whom you capture as birds. I will also tear off your veils and save My people from your hands, and they will no longer be in your hands as prey; and you will know that I am the LORD'" (Ezekiel 13:20-21).

Then, there is this:

> There are wicked men and women who have perfect [sic] the art of magic and sorcery and are still secretly using them to influence world affairs. But some readers refuse to believe this because the repetition of so-called fictional movies and books have convinced the deceived world that magic and sorcery are the stuff of make-believe, folklore and fantasy, hardly anything that can happen for real. Such people not only are not Christians, but have allowed themselves to be blinded

to the power of God and, on a lower level, Satan. Do not allow Satan to compartmentalize your mind into thinking that fiction and nonfiction are two distinct areas of human reality. The Lord does not sanction such principles. The only true duality is between those who believe in Jesus Christ, and those who do not. (https://believersweb.org/the-truth-about-magic-witchcraft-and-sorcery/)

In the Acts of the Apostles, God decries the use of magic by those invoking the powerful name of Jesus:

God was performing extraordinary miracles by the hands of Paul, so that handkerchiefs or aprons were even carried from his body to the sick, and the diseases left them and the evil spirits went out. But also some of the Jewish exorcists, who went from place to place, attempted to use the name of the Lord Jesus over those who had the evil spirits, saying, "I order you in the name of Jesus whom Paul preaches!" Now there were seven sons of Sceva, a Jewish chief priest, doing this. But the evil spirit responded and said to them, "I recognize Jesus, and I know of Paul, but who are you?"

And the man in whom was the evil spirit, pounced on them and subdued all of them and overpowered them, so that they fled out of that house naked and wounded. This became known to all who lived in Ephesus, both Jews and Greeks; and fear fell upon them all and the name of the Lord Jesus was being magnified. Also many of those who had believed kept coming, confessing and disclosing their practices. And many of those who practiced magic brought their books together and began burning them in the sight of everyone; and they added up the prices of the books and found it to be fifty thousand pieces of silver. So the word of the Lord was growing and prevailing mightily (Acts 19:11-20).

We could say that the sons of Sceva did not have the right to use the name of Jesus, because they had no real personal connection to Him. In the same pattern, there are many people – many churchgoers – who will perish in hell because they have no personal relationship with Jesus Christ. They only know "the Jesus the pastor preaches" or "the Jesus my spouse believes in" instead of the Jesus of their own salvation." (https://enduringword.com/bible-commentary/acts-19)

Satan focused his hateful treachery on the Apostles, using a magician in Samaria named Simon:

Now a man named Simon had previously been practicing magic in the city and astonishing the people of Samaria, claiming to be someone great; and all the people, from small to great, were paying attention to him, saying, "This man is the Power of God that is called Great." And they were paying attention to him because for a long time he had astounded them with his magic arts" (Acts 8:9-11).

Even after hearing the true gospel of Jesus, and choosing to be baptized, Simon still did not understand and thought he could buy the gift of the Holy Spirit from Peter and John:

Then they began laying their hands on them, and they were receiving the Holy Spirit. Now when Simon saw that the Spirit was given through the laying on of the apostles' hands, he offered them money, saying, "Give this authority to me as well, so that everyone on whom I lay my hands may receive the Holy Spirit." But Peter said to him, "May your silver perish with you, because you thought you could acquire the gift of God with money! You have no part or share in this matter, for your heart is not right before God. Therefore, repent of this wickedness of yours, and pray to the Lord that, if possible, the intention of your heart will be forgiven you. For I see that you are in the gall of bitterness and in the bondage of unrighteousness." But Simon answered and said, "Pray to the Lord for me yourselves, so that nothing of what you have said may come upon me" (Acts 8:17-24).

Peter, the Apostle, refuted Simon, telling him that the Holy Spirit is only given by faith. Peter explained to Simon how the Holy Spirit cannot be purchased, the powers of the Holy Spirit cannot be bought. Simon the Sorcerer was incensed, convinced Peter was lying to him. Simon seized the opportunity to gather his own followers, wowing them with his magical wonders:

> The false religious system began very early almost with Pentecost in 31 A.D. Even in the earliest of Paul's epistles, he informs us that "the mystery of iniquity DOTH ALREADY WORK" (II Thess. 2:7). Paul wrote this in 50 or 51 AD. The plot to supplant the Truth had already begun. In the later epistles of Paul and in those of the other Apostles, we find it gaining considerable momentum. However, even though the Apostles discuss the diabolical system which was arising, THEY NOWHERE MENTION HOW IT STARTED. They had no need in mentioning its beginning, that had already been done!

> The book of Acts is the KEY to the understanding of Christian beginnings. Not only does it show the commencement of the TRUE Church, but it equally reveals the origins of the False Church masquerading as Christianity. Indeed, you would think it odd if the book of Acts did not discuss this vital subject. (https:// archangel16.livejournal.com/180135.html)

Further proof:

> After the ascension of Yeshua Messiah (Jesus Christ), Simon Peter (Kepha) left Jerusalem BRIEFLY to travel

to Samaria, and then RETURNED to Jerusalem. Simon Magus met Simon Peter in Samaria and later went on to usurp Christianity under Catholicism. Simon Peter traveled to the places he wrote of (Pontus, Galatia, Cappadocia, Asia, and Bithynia), but never mentioned traveling to Rome (1 Peter 1:1). Peter NEVER served as the first pope of the Catholic Church or the bishop of Rome.

Simon Magus went on to deceive many, founding Roman Catholicism, usurping Simon Peter's name, and declaring Himself God on Earth and the first Catholic pope. Simon Peter returned to Jerusalem and remained there to be the apostle to the Jews (Acts 8:25; Galatians 2:7-8). (http://scripturetruthministries. com/2018/03/26/catholicisms-first-pope-simon-magus/)

Many other religions sprang from Simon's church in Rome. We can see how Satan was busy causing divisions to skew our Christ Jesus' message of salvation from the start, spilling debauchery and deceit into the heart of new Christian worship and fellowship.

Our Creator made it clear that His Holy Spirit is for believers, and cannot be used as part of a "magic act."

This passage has caused much controversy. It's meaning, nonetheless, is understandable in its simplicity:

On this rock I will build My church: The words "this rock" have been the source of much controversy. It is best to see them as referring to either Jesus Himself (perhaps Jesus gesturing to Himself as He said this), or as referring to Peter's confession of who Jesus is.

    i.   Peter, by His own testimony, did not see *himself* as the rock on which the church was founded. He wrote that we are living stones, but Jesus is the cornerstone. We could say that Peter was the "first believer"; that he was the "first rock" among "many rocks."

ii.   Peter said as much in 1 Peter 2:4-5: *Coming to Him as to a living stone, rejected indeed by men, but chosen by God and precious, you also, as living stones, are being built up a spiritual house, a holy priesthood, to offer up spiritual sacrifices acceptable to God through Jesus Christ."* (https://enduringword.com/bible-commentary/matthew-16/)

The exchange between Jesus and Peter incontestably does not establish an earthly church, as Satan would want us to think. Rather, Jesus was making a clear claim of ownership of His heavenly church for believers on earth, calling it "My Church."

The Church, His Church, the Body of Believers, belongs to Him, to Jesus.

Chapter Eighteen

The Enemy Wants Your Soul

Dirty Tricks

The book of Hebrews 5:1-4 describes in detail the scope and duties of the office of high priest. These verses describe the differences between the high priests of the old covenant and our Christ Jesus, the new and forever High Priest of the new covenant. Hebrews 5:5-10 tells us that God appointed Jesus to this divine office.

God clearly established there would be no nonsense within His newly established church, appointing Jesus as the High Priest. Jesus knew what it was like to be tempted; recall how Satan tempted Him in the desert in the book of Luke 4:1-13.

Jesus openly revealed His full humanity. He was hungry from fasting, and He most likely was tired, too. His remarkable ability to resist temptation was clearly shown; He had the power to tell Satan to "be gone." Jesus was tempted, He did not succumb. He remained sinless. During His struggles with Satan, Jesus quoted God's Word, and fought the enemy's traps.

Satan was trying to trap and own Jesus' soul. The purpose for tempting Jesus was to lure Him, conquer Him, and thus enjoy the most critical victory over God. Since Jesus was fully God and fully human, and therefore able to sympathize with the reality of temptation, Satan had to have believed Jesus would yield to the desires of the flesh.

Satan has been working relentlessly, since God created man, to bring mankind into outright rebellion to God's authority. We saw this in the Garden of Eden, through the days of Noah, the rebellion in the city of Babel, and into the present time.

Satan rules the earth and has been having his way with humanity. Sin truly is a spiritual disease that spreads easily. Satan's immense pride raises him up at the expense of all others, getting immense pleasure in seeing God's children suffer. Evil penetrates the heart of man, welcoming sinful ways into their lives over and over, oblivious to the consequences.

There are those who mistakenly believe Satan is God's evil equal, embracing a yin-yang philosophy, an Eastern approach to life dating back to the third century BC. The Yin-yang concept in Eastern thought incorporates two complementary opposite and equal forces that make up all aspects of life.

This simply is not true.

> Satan is not omnipresent, he can't be present everywhere at the same time. When you are tempted, or attacked by Satan it may not be Satan himself, it is most likely one of his fallen angels or demons. Along with that, he is not omnipotent. While he does have power, and is truly powerful, he is not all-powerful. There are limits to his power and ability. You should also note that he is not omniscient. He may know a lot, but he does not know everything. He is not equivalent with God. As God would say it,
>
> *Remember the former things, those of long ago; I am God, and there is no other; I am God, and there is none like me.* – Isaiah 46:9-10
>
> I don't know if you have ever heard someone say "the devil is a liar." Usually, we say that with a little jest in the tone. But why do we even say that? Because Satan *is* a liar. Look at what Jesus said about Satan:
>
> *You belong to your father, the devil, and you want to carry out your father's desires. He was a murderer from the beginning, not holding to the truth, for there is no truth in him. When he lies, he speaks his native language, for he is a liar and the father of lies.* – John 8:44
>
> Satan only speaks one language, the language of lies. In fact, he is incapable of speaking truth because as Jesus said *there is no truth in him*. Everything about his influence in this earth is all about lying. It started with Adam and Eve in the garden, and it continues now.

Satan works in the art of deception. He works hard to get you to believe something that is not true. I heard someone say that one of his greatest deceptions is trying to convince people he doesn't exist. When people believe something to be true they will often respond to that truth with their words and actions.

When you consider many of the cults, false teachings, and false belief systems that exist in our society, they all flow out of Satanic deception. I believe this is his greatest work in the hearts of men. He wants to keep people separated from the truth because as Jesus said, you will know the truth and the truth shall set you free. (John 8:32)

He knows this is his end and what awaits him. His goal, therefore, is to try to take as many people with him as possible into this place that was created for him (Matthew 25:41). That's why we must preach the gospel and proclaim the truth so we can snatch people from the kingdom of darkness and bring them into the kingdom of light.

(https://www.crosswalk.com/faith/bible-study/facts-about-satan-you-need-to-know.html)

Satan is the father of all lies (John 8:44), recruiting people in this way:

Satan and his Demons (The Original Gods) protect us and look out for us as we transform and achieve personal power. With Satan, we have protection that outsiders do not have. We can advance in the powers of the mind and soul as far as we wish. For outsiders, this can prove dangerous. Satan also gives us knowledge.

(https://satanisgod.org/)

Satan knows the Bible backwards and forwards, misquoting or scrambling Scripture in an attempt to destroy someone's faith. A good example of this is an exchange between the enemy and Jesus. When Satan tried to tempt Jesus to throw himself down from the temple roof, he was quoting from Scripture, "If you are the Son of God, throw yourself down, for it is written, 'He will command his angels concerning you'" (Matthew 4:6).

Satan is sneaky. He does not always ruin faith simply by saying, "The Bible isn't true." He more often than not tries to destroy our faith by professing some passage and then using that very passage to lead us into disobedience.

> Jesus called Satan the "prince of all of this world." When Satan offered Jesus all the kingdoms of the world, Jesus did not say, *they are not yours to give* (Luke 4:1-13), because he knew perfectly well they were Satan's to give and it is a horrible thought if you really realize it that the world in which we live is ruled over by Satan, he is the prince of this world, but let's take it a step further, He said he's not only the ruler, or prince of this world, he is the god of this world, the only person besides his heavenly father to whom Jesus ever applied the word god was Satan:

> And even if our gospel is veiled, it is veiled to those who are perishing, in whose case the god of this world has blinded the minds of the unbelieving so that they will not see the light of the gospel of the glory of Christ, who is the image of God. (2 Cor 4:3-4)

> He said my heavenly Father is God of everything, but of this world Satan is god which means very simply not only that Satan controls this world and is able to manipulate science and education and politics for his own ends (Ephesians 6:12).

> More than that Satan is the real god whom most people on earth worship (Matthew 7:13-14) whether they know it or not that behind so much religion, so much activity, Satan is the one who is being worshipped

he's the person and even by some who go to church and chapel on Sunday in reality he's their god (1 Cor 10:20, Matthew 7:21-23) for they worship the things he offers them, they want the things of the world that he belongs to and rules over (1 John 2:15-16) rather than setting their minds on the things that are above where Jesus is (Colossians 2:3).

And if you want this world and if you want the things of this world then I give you a piece of advice, make Satan your god. If you want this world he's a wonderful god to have because he'll give it to you there's always a price to pay when the bill comes in you may not be quite so happy, but he'll give it to you. He can give you money, he can give you fame, he can give you anything you want, because it's his to give.

(https://www.facebook.com/3n1Ministry/ videos/722475555567045)

Satan is not the conclusive authority in the world, and in Luke 4:6, he admits this: "To you I will give all this authority and their glory, for it has been delivered to me." Who delivered this authority to Satan? God did. In his sovereignty, God considered it prudent, as part of the punishment on the world after the fall of Adam and Eve, to give Satan this power in the world. Satan wants to fool you so deeply into believing that you're undeservingly sinful that you can't believe that Jesus sacrificially died for you on the cross.

Satan uses half-truths to trick you. He'll mock you. He'll destroy you if you decide to let him.

Chapter Nineteen

Legions of Demons

Satan's Helpers

Be of sober spirit, be on the alert.
Your adversary, the devil, prowls around like a roaring lion,
seeking someone to devour.

1 Peter 5:8

During a time prior to Genesis 3, Lucifer, a leading angel, rebelled against God and was swiftly judged (Ezekiel 28, Isaiah 14). It is believed many other angels rebelled with him during this time, becoming the fallen angels or demons mentioned throughout the Bible. Lucifer was banished from heaven and was called Satan thereafter.

Although the number is not specified in Scripture, many other angels that followed and adored Lucifer in heaven, also rebelled against God, and were banished, too. Satan does not work alone, and the other fallen angels, called demons, work for him to torment believers (2 Corinthians 12:7).

Satan and his demons can and will inflict harm on earth by entering the bodies of willing persons, ultimately possessing them. Demons bring physical and spiritual harm (Matthew 12:22; Mark 5:1-20), and provoke those whom they dwell within to do evil, as seen in Luke 22:3-4. Demons will blind the minds of unbelievers, and close their spiritual ears to God's voice, so that they cannot see nor can they hear the Gospel (2 Corinthians 4:4).

Satan, the father of lies (John 8:44), and his helpers deceive people into considering themselves as "servants of righteousness" (2 Corinthians 11:14-15). Satan sometimes appears as an "angel of light" (2 Corinthians 11:14); likewise, false apostles can appear to be forthright and above-board, even though they are promoting false doctrine (1 Timothy 4:1), making outlandish claims in order to profit from an enthusiastic and undiscerning following.

Satan and his demonic forces are organized in hierarchical levels known as rulers, authorities, powers, and spiritual forces of evil. "For our struggle is not against flesh and blood, but against the rulers, against the powers, against the world forces of this darkness, against the spiritual forces of wickedness in the heavenly places" (Ephesians 6:12).

People can be demonized which is another term for demonic possession (Luke 8:30).

> They went into Capernaum; and immediately on the
> Sabbath Jesus entered the synagogue and began to
> teach. And they were amazed at His teaching; for
> He was teaching them as one having authority, and
> not as the scribes. Just then there was a man in their
> synagogue with an unclean spirit; and he cried out,
> saying, "What business do you have with us, Jesus of
> Nazareth? Have You come to destroy us? I know who
> You are: the Holy One of God!" And Jesus rebuked
> him, saying, "Be quiet, and come out of him!" After
> throwing him into convulsions and crying out with
> a loud voice, the unclean spirit came out of him.
> And they were all amazed, so they debated among
> themselves, saying, "What is this? A new teaching with
> authority! He commands even the unclean spirits, and
> they obey Him" (Mark 1:21-27).

Referencing the above Scripture verses, notice how Jesus taught his disciples how to cast out demons:

> Jesus rebuked him: Jesus didn't need to rely on hocus-
> pocus or ceremonies. He simply demonstrated the
> authority of God.

> Be quiet: Jesus often told demons to shut up. Today,
> many self-styled deliverers from demon possession
> encourage the demons to speak, or even *believe* what
> the demons say. Jesus avoided such theatrics and
> merely delivered the afflicted man.

> Be quiet, and come out of him! There were other
> exorcists in Jesus' day. He was not the only one
> who tried to cast out demons. But there was a huge
> difference between Jesus and other exorcists. They
> used long, fancy, elaborate, superstitious ceremonies

and they often failed. Jesus never failed to cast out a demon, and He never used an elaborate ceremony.

(https://enduringword.com/bible-commentary/ mark-1/)

Jesus assigned his apostles to preach and cast out demons, "And He appointed twelve, so that they would be with Him and that He could send them out to preach, and to have authority to cast out the demons" (Mark 3:14-15), and this, "Behold, I have given you authority to walk on snakes and scorpions, and authority over all the power of the enemy, and nothing will injure you" (Luke 10:19), and this, "Jesus summoned His twelve disciples and gave them authority over unclean spirits, to cast them out, and to heal every disease and every sickness" (Matthew 10:1).

Jesus continued to teach,

So why does it seem demons will obey some believers and not others? Because our authority is accessed through faith. Jesus gave His disciples authority over ALL powers of the enemy (Luke 10:19), but when they reached a demon they couldn't cast out, He told them it was because of their unbelief, as we can see in Matthew 17:19-20: "Then came the disciples to Jesus apart, and said, Why could not we cast him out? And Jesus said unto them, Because of your unbelief."

Jesus went on to say that some demons are so strong and stubborn, that prayer and fasting is required to drive them out, Matthew 17:21: "Howbeit this kind goeth not out but by prayer and fasting." Prayer and fasting builds up your faith like nothing else and sometimes it's necessary to drive out the stronger demons. The more faith you have, the more authority you'll be able to exercise against demonic spirits. (http://www.ministeringdeliverance.com/who_ cast_demons.php)

Scripture clearly states how followers of our Christ Jesus have authority over Satan, demons, fallen angels, rulers, principalities and powers through the power of His Holy Name. "Hell is a real place, made by God for Satan and his angels. If humans choose to serve Satan in this life, then they will dwell eternally with Satan in Hell (Matthew 8:12, 25:46, 1 Thessalonians 1:9)" (*Systematic Theology Outline*, 1990, p. 147).

Jesus goes into great detail to describe what is obviously an actual eye-witness account in Luke 16:19-31 to fully describe hell and the torment that awaits those who do not accept His offered salvation. It is described as a place of great torment in both the Old and New Testaments.

Satan originated sin in the universe and is the person responsible for it (Ezekiel 28:12-17). "The difference between Satan's fall and mankind's fall is that Satan fell without any external tempter and as such, can never be redeemed" (*Systematic Theology Outline*, 1990, p. 150).

> Can believers be demon inhabited? This is a question which many ask. Theologically considered, it is hard to believe that it is possible that a believer can both be a dwelling place for a demon and the temple of the indwelling Holy Spirit (1 Cor. 6:19 and 2 Cor. 6:16). However, there is every reason to believe that a believer may be demonized in the sense of being oppressed by demonic malevolence (1 Pet 5:8-9). Likewise, the devil may actively seek to harass a godly servant as Paul tells the Corinthians (2 Cor. 12:7). In brief: inhabited, no; oppressed, yes.
>
> https://www.crossway.org/articles/10-things-you-should-know-about-demons/)

Any power Satan has is permitted by God. He can only do certain things. He is permitted to afflict the righteous (Job 1:12), he is allowed to have sinners under his dominion (Acts 26:18), he can veil the minds of the unbelievers (2 Corinthians 4:3-4), and he can do counterfeit miracles (2 Thessalonians 2:9).

However, Satan is limited by Divine authority (Luke 10:19, Romans 16:20), he is limited in the scope of his temptations (1 Corinthians 10:13), in his power over believers (James 4:7), and in his time before further judgment (Revelation 12:12, 13:5). Satan is the grand deceiver who attempts to ruin men and women by lying promises, twisting God's Word, and appearing as an angel of light.

Demons cannot create a person within to dwell, although they can and will attempt to control believers, tormenting their minds and emotions, through their God-given gift of free will. God does not permit them to abide in a believer's spirit and they cannot control anyone's will (Mark 5:1-6). The *person* has to *decide*.

Followers of Jesus, our Christ, have been given the power by God to use over demonic powers. Every true believer has authority over demons and should not be intimidated by demons or demon-possessed people.

Satan and his minions have been busy corrupting men and women in this world since the fall of mankind in the Garden of Eden. After our Christ Jesus' death and resurrection, Satan's full fury was unleashed on earth.

One thousand years after He ascended into heaven, the world was filled with debauchery from the spoils of sin. Promises of power and earthly riches have always been used as lures by Satan and his minions to capture souls.

As time progressed, Satan's tricks and treachery became more and more obvious to those with "ears to hear and eyes to see" (Matthew 6:22-23).

Chapter Twenty

The Stage Is Set

Using People, Places, and Things

A few years ago, while in the midst of prayer, I realized I no longer could pray for Israel and the Jewish people. I felt like a heretic, a phony, a babble-mouth spewing words when I did. I knew I was supposed to pray for Israel. Yet, the words were not coming from my heart. God's so-called chosen people sure seemed to be engaging in a lot of criminal activity.

So, of course, I went to God's Throne to ask Him about this problem I was having. How could I pray for the gangsters in charge of the Federal Reserve, knowing they were stealing from us and committing usury? How could I pray for people who were intentionally lying about God's creation, those who were poisoning our food on purpose and tainting our waterways? How could I pray for a country so rife with debauchery that its capital of Tel Aviv is known as the "gayest city on earth"? (https://www.bostonglobe.com/lifestyle/travel/2016/03/17/welcome-tel-aviv-gayest-city-earth/y9V15VazXhtSjXVSo9gT9K/story.html)

How in God's world could I pray for the liars at NASA, spending billions of tax dollars on space scams. Yes, of course I pray for my enemies; however, it seemed as though most of my greater oppressors were calling themselves Jewish.

Then, He spoke to me in a dream. Jesus told me to pray for His family and His beloved homeland. After all, He will be returning to rule over the earth from there. He understood my dilemma and told me to investigate the Truth. So, I did.

Tracing history from the fall of the Roman empire through the Crusades, to the present time does not need to be done to expose the evils in this world. Most people are aware of the carnage during this time period, much has been written about it. This book is an historical account of how Satan's magic and sorcery have caused chaos.

Magnifying an obscure, rarely talked about civilization, Satan's sinister plans to plunge the earth's inhabitants into hell with him becomes evident. This ancient civilization heavily influences our lives today, even though very few people know about it.

Recall how Isaac blessed Jacob instead of Esau under false pretenses in the book of Genesis. Isaac blessed his son and said:

> "Surely, the smell of my son
> Is like the smell of a field
> Which the LORD has blessed.
> Therefore may God give you
> Of the dew of heaven,
> Of the fatness of the earth,
> And plenty of grain and wine.
> Let peoples serve you,
> And nations bow down to you.
> Be master over your brethren,
> And let your mother's sons bow down to you.
> Cursed be everyone who curses you,
> And blessed be those who bless you!" (Genesis 27:27-29)

James Montgomery Boice, Bible teacher, author, and international speaker on the topics of scriptural authority and inerrancy, comments on these verses,

> **And blessed him**: Isaac blessed Jacob as the spiritual head of the family. *Isaac* had the right (not Ishmael) to pass on this blessing related to the covenant of Abraham. The son (Jacob or Esau) who received this blessing was able to pass it on to his descendants.

> **May God give you of the dew of heaven, of the fatness of the earth**: The words of the blessing were filled with pictures of the LORD's rich bounty, and they echoed some of the words of the covenant God made with Abraham.

> **Cursed be everyone who curses you, and blessed be those who bless you**: Again, it is important to see it wasn't the bestowal of these words upon Jacob that

made him blessed. Instead, Jacob was blessed because God chose him long before (Genesis 25:23). What mattered was that *God* said *the older shall serve the younger* (back in Genesis 25:23), not that *Isaac* said **be master over your brethren.**

i. "The point is that the sovereign will of God is done, in spite of our or any other person's opposition to it." (Boice)

(https://enduringword.com/bible-commentary/genesis-27/)

This blessing of Jacob profoundly impacted the sociological and geological structure of the world. The spiritual storm that followed is evident to this day.

This is what happened:

> Edomites are therefore descended from Edom (Esau) whose descendants later intermarried with the Turks to produce a Turco-Edomite mixture which later became known as Khazars. That is, most of today's Jews are descendants of this interbreeding that produced a race called Khazars who had once governed an empire called Khazaria. Furthermore, this hybrid race Edomite/Turk/Khazar who created the Khazar kingdom and who between the seventh and ninth centuries AD, adopted the religion of Judaism. And, it is these Khazar Jews who are the ancestors of the vast majority of today's Jewish people. That is, Edomite/Turk/Khazars are the ancestors of the modern "Jews" including the Torah-true and Zionist Jews who spuriously claim right to the land of Palestine claiming it it [*sic*] is theirs by biblical demands and ancestral rights.

> Consequently, the majority of today's Jewish people are known as "Jews" not because they are Judahites and descended from Jacob/Israel but because their

Edomite/Turk/Khazar ancestors in their Kingdom
of Khazaria adopted the religion of Judaism, called
themselves "Jews" and arrogated the Birthright
Promises and Bible Covenants belonging to the
Israelites, but especially those belonging to the
Judahites.

Thus, "Jews" are *not* Israelites and certainly they are
not Judahites. Hence, modern Jews are *not* heir to the
Bible Covenants nor to the ancient Nation of Israel
given by Yahweh to the Israelites and the Judahites
and so have no Divine Right or biblical mandate to the
modern Land of Palestine.

(https://www.jewworldorder.org/history-khazarians-
todays-jews/)

Here is the fascinating timeline of events. Patching this together
from an historical point of view, we see a fabric of debauchery woven
from the Serpent himself. Ancient Khazaria occupied the land in an
area roughly known today as Ukraine. Between the years of 100 and
800 AD, an incredibly evil society emerged in Khazaria.

Khazarians develop into a nation ruled by an evil
king, who had ancient Babylonian black arts, occult
oligarchs serving as his court. During this time,
Khazarians became known to surrounding countries
as thieves, murderers, road bandits, and for assuming
the identities of those travelers they murdered as a
normal occupational practice and way of life. (https://
geopolitics.co/2015/03/11/hidden-history-of-the-
incredibly-evil-khazarian-mafia/)

Sometime around the year 800 AD, an ultimatum was delivered to
the Khazarians by Russia and other surrounding nations:

The leaders of the surrounding nations, especially
Russia, have had so many years of complaints by their
citizens that, as a group, they deliver an ultimatum

to the Khazarian king. They send a communique to the Khazarian king that he must choose one of the three Abrahamic religions for his people, make it his official state religion and require all Khazarian citizens to practice it, and socialize all Khazarian children to practice that faith.

The Khazarian king was given a choice between Islam, Christianity and Judaism. The Khazarian king chose Judaism, and promised to stay within the requirements laid out by the surrounding confederacy of nations led by the Russian czar. Despite his agreement and promise, the Khazarian king and his inner circle of oligarchs kept practicing ancient Babylonian black-magic, also known as Secret Satanism. This Secret Satanism involved occult ceremonies featuring child sacrifice, after "bleeding them out", drinking their blood and eating their hearts.

The deep dark secret of the occult ceremonies was that they were all based on ancient Baal Worship, also known as worship of the Owl. In order to fool the confederacy of nations led by Russia that were watching Khazaria, the Khazarian king melded these Luciferian black-magick practices with Judaism and created a secret Satanic-hybrid religion known as Babylonian Talmudism. This was made the national religion of Khazaria, and nurtured the same evil that Khazaria was known for before.

Sadly, the Khazarians continued their evil ways, robbing and murdering those from surrounding countries who traveled through Khazaria.

Khazarian robbers often attempted to assume their identities after they murdered these visitors, and became masters of disguises and false identities a practice they have continued even to this very day, along with their child-sacrifice occult ceremonies, which are actually ancient Baal Worship. (https:// www.veteranstoday.com/2022/03/10/the-hidden-history-of-the-incredibly-evil-khazarian-mafia/)

By the year 1200 AD, Russia and the surrounding nations had had enough and took action:

> About 1,200 [*sic*] AD, the Russians led a group of nations surrounding Khazaria and invaded it, in order to stop the Khazarian crimes against their people, which included kidnapping of their young children and infants for their blood sacrifice ceremonies to Baal. The Khazarian king and his inner court of criminals and murderers came to be known as the Khazarian Mafia (KM) by neighboring countries.

> The Khazarian leaders had a well-developed spy network through which they obtained prior warning and escaped from Khazaria to European nations to the west, taking their vast fortune with them in gold and silver. They laid low and regrouped, while assuming new identities. In secret, they continued their Satanic child blood and sacrifice rituals, and trusted Baal to give them the whole world and all its riches, as they claimed he had promised them, as long as they kept bleeding out and sacrificing children and infants for him.

> The Khazarian king and his court Mafia plotted eternal revenge against the Russians and the surrounding nations that invaded Khazaria and drove them from power. (https://www.veteranstoday. com/2022/03/10/the-hidden-history-of-the-incredibly-evil-khazarian-mafia/)

Keeping in mind God has allowed Satan to rule the earth for now, this patchwork quilt of history helps us to understand the conflict and strife in today's world. The history of this region is outlined in the book shown in the beginning of the quote below:

> The Thirteenth Tribe: The Khazar Empire and its Heritage
>
> All original editions. Nothing added, nothing removed. This book traces the history of the ancient Khazar Empire, a major but almost forgotten power in Eastern Europe, which in the Dark Ages became converted to Judaism. Khazaria was finally wiped out by the forces of Genghis Khan, but evidence indicates that the Khazars themselves migrated to Poland and formed the cradle of Western Jewry. To the general reader the Khazars, who flourished from the 7th to 11th century, may seem infinitely remote today. Yet they have a close and unexpected bearing on our world, which emerges as Koestler recounts the fascinating history of the ancient Khazar Empire. At about the time that Charlemagne was Emperor in the West. The Khazars' sway extended from the Black Sea to the Caspian, from the Caucasus to the Volga, and they were instrumental in stopping the Muslim onslaught against Byzantium, the eastern jaw of the gigantic pincer movement that in the West swept across northern Africa and into Spain. Thereafter the Khazars found themselves in a precarious position between the two major world powers: the Eastern Roman Empire in Byzantium and the triumphant followers of Mohammed. As Koestler points out, the Khazars were the Third World of their day. They chose a surprising method of resisting both the Western pressure to become Christian and the Eastern to adopt Islam. Rejecting both, they converted to Judaism. Mr. Koestler speculates about the ultimate faith of the Khazars and their impact on the racial composition and social heritage of modern Jewry.
>
> (https://www.amazon.com/Thirteenth-Tribe-

Khazar)

In 1917 the Khazarians got their revenge.

When studying the 1917 invasion of Russia Whites
refer to the Russians or Russian people who were loyal
to Russia and Reds refer to the red Russian Khazarian
Communist Jews.

All the evil, all the mass murdering of the USSR was not
done by White Russians.

It was done by Jews. Khazarian Communist Jews.
The Khazarian Jew Joseph Stalin who Holocausted
an estimated 66 million humans. Of those, around 13
million were Ukrainians. The Khazarian Jew Stalin
Holocausted an estimated 13 million Ukrainians ...
using rape/murder and starvation. He then replaced
the Ukrainians with Russians, more than likely
meaning Khazarian Jews.

During WW 2 many Ukrainians served with the
Germans against the USSR not because of loyalty to
Germany, but because it was the only game in town to
fight for their freedom from the Khazarian Jews who
had mass murdered their people and families.

Many White Russians and Cossacks served in/under
the German army against the Khazarian Jews of the
USSR. This was not adhering to Germany's cause or
believes [*sic*], it was an attempt to become free of the
Khazarian Jews running Russia.

The history of WW 1 & WW 2 is long and convoluted
but Germany did not start either war as you have been
told, Germany wanted neither war. Germany in WW2
wanted to be free of the Khazarian Jews which had
been put in charge of Germany after Germany's defeat
in WW1 facilitated by treason of Khazarian Jews

living in Germany. (https://www.jewworldorder.org/
bit-of-khazarian-history-in-relation-to-the-takeover-
of-russia-by-the-khazarians-in-1917-with-continuing-
ramifications-today/)

So, we can see how the wealthy Rothschilds orchestrated the start of both wars against Germany from their strongholds in Washington, DC, and London. Nathan Rothschild said,

> "I care not what puppet is placed upon the throne of England to rule the empire on which the sun never sets. The man who controls Britain's money supply controls the British empire, and I control the British money supply"
>
> (https://www.donaldwatkins.com/post/the-rothschilds-controlling-the-world-s-money-supply-for-more-than-two-centuries).

The Khazarian Jews resumed their ancient role of running the Khazarian region, now called Ukraine. The Rothschilds are oblivious to the hierarchy of the Khazarian Jews. They simply use them for their own purposes to gain more wealth and control. The Rothschilds, who own and control Palestine, used the Khazarian Jews to keep wars going. They all lie to each other and use each other, bringing starstruck minions into their fold by promising them outrageous wealth and power.

> It is becoming public knowledge the Khazarian Jews who have no legitimate or heritage claim to Palestine as they are not descended from Biblical Hebrews from occupied Palestine along with the Khazarian Jews running Washington DC did 9-11, the Khazarian Jews in Palestine have stopped being a useful tool and become a liability to the Rothschilds. So, they are killing off the Khazarian jews in Palestine." (https://www.johnccarleton.org/BLOGGER/2022/02/27/

bit-of-khazarian-history-in-relation-to-the-takeover-
of-russia-by-the-khazarians-in-1917/)

Hold onto your hat for this one:

> Who should possess the land of Israel? Christian
> evangelicals say it should be the descendants of
> Abraham. They point to the Old Testament and claim
> that God gave this land forever to the descendants of
> Abraham and that God demands they and they alone
> own the land. To the Christian evangelical, this means
> the Jews. Yes, it is the Jews who own this land, and
> it is their land forever. The Jews, then, according
> to Christian evangelicals, are the descendants of
> Abraham, his *seed.*
>
> There is only one problem. And it is a huge one.
> Science proves those who call themselves "Jews" are
> *not* Jews! *DNA Science has confounded the Christian
> evangelicals by proving conclusively that most of the
> people in the nation of Israel and in World Jewry are
> not the descendants of Abraham.*
>
> Those living today who profess to be "Jews" are *not*
> of the ancient Israelites, and they are *not* the seed of
> Abraham. In fact, the new DNA research shows that the
> Palestinians actually have more Israelite blood than do
> the "Jews!"
>
> The nation of Israel today is populated with seven and
> half [*sic*] million *imposters.* The "Jews" Are Not Jews
> But Are Khazarians.
>
> (https://educate yourself.org/cn/
> texemarrskhazarianjews08mar13.shtml)

The Khazarian Mafia is a Satanic group claiming personal
partnership with Baal, also known as Moloch, a god of Canaanite
origin, just as the evil kings in the Old Testament did.

They are Satanists. They perform child sacrifices and engage in Satanic rituals to placate Baal/Moloch. They hate any kings, presidents, or leaders who rule under the authority of God.

> In the 1600's, the KM (Khazarian Mafia) murder the British Royals and substitute their own fakes. In the 1700s, they murder the French Royals. Right before WWI [*sic*] they murder Austrian Archduke Ferdinand to start WW1. In 1917 they assembled [*sic*] their KM army, the Bolsheviks, and infiltrate and hijack Russia, murder the Czar and his family in cold blood, bayoneted his favorite daughter through the chest and steal all the Russian gold, silver and art treasures. Right before WW2, they murder the Austrian and German Royals. Then they get rid of the Chinese Royals and disempower the Japanese ruler.
>
> The Khazarian Mafia's intense hatred of anyone who professed faith in any God but their god Baal has motivated them to murder kings and royalty, and make sure they can never rule. They have done the same with American presidents running sophisticated covert operations to disempower them.
>
> If that doesn't work the Khazarian Mafia assassinates them, like they did to McKinley, Lincoln and JFK. The Khazarian Mafia wants to eliminate any strong rulers or elected officials who dare to resist their Babylonian money-magick power or their covert power gained from their deployment of their human compromise network."

(https://geopolitics.co/2015/03/11/hidden-history-of-the-incredibly-evil-khazarian-mafia/)

Satan has always flaunted in full disclosure how he works and what he's doing right in front of us, mocking us for not noticing. The precious gift of free will to discover and decide is tossed aside, instead, choosing to blindly accept Satan's spurious, deceitful activity due to laziness and complacency.

> The history of the Khazarians, specifically the
> Khazarian Mafia (KM), the World's largest Organized
> Crime Syndicate that the Khazarian oligarchy morphed
> into by their deployment of Babylonian Money-Magick,
> has been nearly completely excised from the history
> books.
>
> The present day KM knows that it cannot operate or
> exist without abject secrecy, and therefore has spent a
> lot of money having its history excised from the history
> books in order to prevent citizens of the World from
> learning about its "Evil beyond imagination", that
> empowers this World's largest Organized Crime Cabal.
>
> (https://geopolitics.co/2015/03/11/hidden-
> history-of-the-incredibly-evil-khazarian-mafia/)

The Deceiver recreated the State of Israel using the Edomites, the Khazarians, who are the descendants of Esau, to attempt to take down God's creation. Satan's intention all along was to corrupt and ruin God's precious children and destroy God's world through his hateful, evil manipulations.

Next, we will explore just how deep and broad Satan's work has been, infiltrating every corner of the earth. Madness, mayhem and chaos reign, causing confusion, striking fear into the hearts of God's children.

Behold, I will make those of the synagogue of Satan,
who say that they are Jews and are not, but lie—
I will make them come and bow down before your feet,
and make them know that I have loved you.
Revelation 3:9

– End of Part Two –

PART THREE

What It Is Like Today

Trust in the LORD with all your heart
And do not lean on your own understanding.
Proverbs 3:5

Dear Lord God Almighty,

Creator of Everything,

Please show me Your Truth,

And hold me up when I faint.

Thank You.

Amen

Chapter Twenty-One
Creation in Chaos

Who Are These People?

I know where you dwell, where Satan's throne is; and you hold firmly to My name, and did not deny My faith even in the days of Antipas, My witness, My faithful one, who was killed among you, where Satan dwells.

Revelation 2:13

Indeed, two of the biggest lies of the last century are these: Hell doesn't exist and Satan is not real. The tricksters, minions of Satan himself, want us to believe God is nothing more than a mostly benevolent, on occasion dreadfully terrible, character in fairy tales. The world which God has allowed Satan to roam free seems to have succumbed to the mind-numbing disease of obliviousness, its peoples believing what they are told rather than thinking for themselves.

Satan's laughter echoes across the earth as God's precious gift of free will is nearly obliterated, barely recognizable under the dirty pile of the devil's deceptions. Men and women draw conclusions from what they are told rather than listening for the call of their Creator.

> As we received mercy, we do not lose heart, but we have renounced the things hidden because of shame, not walking in trickery nor distorting the word of God, but by the open proclamation of the truth commending ourselves to every person's conscience in the sight of God. And even if our gospel is veiled, it is veiled to those who are perishing, in whose case the god of this world has blinded the minds of the unbelieving so that they will not see the light of the gospel of the glory of Christ, who is the image of God" (2 Cor 4:1-4).

Satan seems to have succeeded in duping most of mankind. The devil no longer is a perceived threat. Instead, the pinnacle of evil itself has morphed himself into a play toy. "The devil made me do it," the excuse for bad behavior, the ultimate battle cry of innocence in the slanguage of sleepy sinners.

Safekeep your hardcover Bibles and books, because Internet searches will tell you the Bible is a bunch of hooey filled with myths. The attempt to cancel God is evident online and all over our secular world. Two thousand years of recorded time recently has changed. Satan has concocted a new way to keep track of time to exclude God. BC and AD were the time measurements used for centuries, until now:

> Understanding where BC and AD came from and why they're used can help make their meanings clear. Together, they form what is known as "the Christian Era." The abbreviation BC stands for "Before Christ." It refers to all time before the theoretical birth of Jesus Christ. The abbreviation AD stands for "*Anno Domini*" in Latin. In English, this means "in the year of our Lord." This abbreviation refers to all time after the theoretical birth of Jesus Christ. AD time starts when BC time ends, but there is no year 0. So, BC starts in the year 1 BC and AD starts in the year AD 1.
>
> (https://abbreviations.yourdictionary.com/articles/ what-do-bc-and-ad-stand-for-dates-in-history.html)

Please take note of the phrase they've used, the "theoretical birth of Jesus Christ."

So, for over 2,000 years, time was measured according to the birth of the world's Savior, Jesus. The oldest, continuously mass-produced book is The Torah, which refers to the first five books of the Bible known as the Old Testament, published in 1312 BC. Yet, here we are, 2,000 years later, changing historical timelines by using BCE, Before Common Era and CE, Common Era, instead of AD.

The perpetrator of lies, the Father of Deception (John 8:44), tempts and we sin. Hell is real. Satan is real, and so are his demons. Teachers who teach lies and preachers who preach lies will be held accountable, whether they believe their own lies or not. There is only one Truth. The Truth is found in God's Word.

Satan has enlisted minions in this world who are hard at work dragging unsuspecting souls into their web of tyranny and deceit. The devil has promised them the ultimate deception, dominion over this world with him. Fame and money at their fingertips, they are hard at work seducing God's children, beckoning them to enter into their web:

> But temptation, getting my way, and obtaining what I want never *feel* like the doorway to tyranny. "Most of the time temptation begins with something good: food, rest, God-approved sex, the need to be loved and accepted." We could go on. Perhaps this is why the first sensation is always one of anticipation, of potential happiness and of greater personal fulfillment. Right? The mind controlled by lust, by *epithumia* (the New Testament Greek word for "strong desires or passions"), has an infinite capacity for rationalization. Let me call to mind here some bits of common thinking, a few thoughts we have all used at one point or another: ...
>
> God wants me to be happy. This makes me happy at the core of my being. How can this be wrong? ...
>
> The people who do not approve of what I am doing are just judgmental nags they make me sick! They are worse than I am! ...
>
> *I am my desires.* Or *I will be the real me when my desires are fulfilled.*
>
> But that kind of life is heartbreaking and delusional. Giving into our desires only strengthens them. This is positive news if the desires are good and holy. It's one of the ways we grow in the grace of God. But if the desires are out of whack, our disordered desire takes greater and greater control of our lives, and we can fall farther and farther into sin.
>
> (https://faithgateway.com/blogs/christian-books/ our-top-five-temptations/)

Clergy rarely talk about sin anymore. Churches operate as businesses; words from the top of the business model are aimed at keeping the congregants happy so they keep coming back. Church expenses are deductible, donations are deductible, false gospels are spoken as long as the pews stay full. Oh, sure, they'll throw in a Scripture here and there to make it seem legit, even though week after week the mark is missed. Half-truths abound, outright lies are spoken. Nonsense reigns, spirituality corrupted. Prolific Christian writer, C. S. Lewis wrote this in *The Screwtape Letters*, "Nonsense in the intellect reinforces corruption in the will." (2016, p. 116)

Jerry Bridges, in his 9-week small-group curriculum study guide, *Respectable Sins,* has this to say, "The very word 'sin,' which seems to have disappeared, was once a proud word. It was once a strong word, an ominous and serious word ... but the word went away. It has almost disappeared, the word along with the notion. Why? Doesn't anyone sin anymore? Doesn't anyone believe in sin?" (Bridges, 2010, p. 14).

Sin, simply, has become passé. It's inconvenient to think about oneself in this world as anything but perfect. God loves us no matter what, right? Isn't that what we've been told in church? Sin is what the bad guys in fairy tales do, we don't do those things. Even if we did, God loves us anyway because we are His pride and joy, right?

The notion of personal responsibility has become uncomfortable, and, in a world filled with creature comforts, the thought of sin has evaporated into a thin air of nothingness.

Satan has been prowling God's earth since his fall from heaven, since the fall of mankind after Satan's seduction of Adam and Eve in the garden. Satan has been busy enlisting the help of humans since Eden. The recruits who have said "yes" to him, the Luciferians, have been busy corrupting God's children in this world for centuries.

Let's explore together what they've done, how they did it, and how we have gotten to this dreadful precipice of destruction.

Chapter Twenty-Two

Corruption of the Corps

Kill Our Body, Our Spirit
Belongs to God

So then, brothers and sisters, we are under obligation,
not to the flesh, to live according to the flesh
for if you are living in accord with the flesh, you are going to die;
but if by the Spirit you are putting to death the deeds of the body, you
will live.

Romans 8:12-13

The Luciferians had to set the stage for destruction subtly, so the people in the world would not notice. Almost magically, certainly deceptively, the food supply in God's perfect creation was tragically altered:

> Genetically modified organisms (GMOs) can be defined as organisms (i.e. plants, animals or microorganisms) in which the genetic material (DNA) has been altered in a way that does not occur naturally by mating and/or natural recombination. The technology is often called "modern biotechnology" or "gene technology", sometimes also "recombinant DNA technology" or "genetic engineering". It allows selected individual genes to be transferred from one organism into another, also between non related species. Foods produced from or using GM organisms are often referred to as GM foods.

> The release of GMOs into the environment and the marketing of GM foods have resulted in a public debate in many parts of the world. This debate is likely to continue, probably in the broader context of other uses of biotechnology (e.g. in human medicine) and their consequences for human societies. (https://www.who.int/news-room/questions-and-answers/item/food-genetically-modified)

Yes, GMOs will make you sick. Here are some findings from government studies completed in 2008:

> Two new government studies, published within days of each other, point to disturbing health hazards of genetically modified (GM) foods.

On November 13th, a study by the Italian National Institute of Research on Food and Nutrition showed how GM corn caused significant immune system changes in mice, related to allergic and inflammatory responses. The corn, sold by Monsanto, contains a gene that produces the toxic "Bt" pesticide in every cell and in every bite. The results raise the question whether this toxin (or some other unpredictable change in the GM corn) might be contributing to the rise in allergies or other immune disorders in North America.

(https://www.huffpost.com/entry/will-genetically-modified_b_145320)

Keep in mind Satan cannot create life; he's doing everything he can to destroy it. Most countries worldwide label foods that contain genetically modified organisms (GMOs).

While the United States and Canada have virtually no GE food labeling laws, countries like Russia, Australia, Italy, and more have mandatory labeling of nearly all GE foods. At this site, you can view a global map of all the countries and their current status with GE labeling laws. (https://www.occupy.com/article/worldwide-gmo-labeling-laws)

The earth's waterways are contaminated, too. This study, from March of 2022, revealed:

A recent York University study of over 250 rivers in over 100 countries around the globe determined that many rivers are contaminated with pharmaceutical drugs. According to the BBC, "more than a quarter of the 258 rivers sampled had what are known as 'active pharmaceutical ingredients' present at a level deemed unsafe for aquatic organisms" (February 15, 2022). The study found high levels of paracetamol (a pain killer), nicotine, caffeine, and drugs used to treat epilepsy and diabetes. How do these chemicals wind up in waterways? Most pass through the bodies of those who use them. Waste treatment plants do not completely break them down, and they are released into the environment.

As the BBC notes, the presence of dissolved human contraceptives has negatively impacted fish development and reproduction, and researchers are concerned that the growing presence of antibiotics in our rivers will increase the level of antibiotic resistance in disease-causing bacteria. The lead author of the study suggests that reducing the availability of antibiotics and other drugs and more restrictive dosages could help begin to solve the problem.

(https://www.tomorrowsworld.org/news-and-prophecy/world-rivers-polluted-with-drugs)

Satan could not stop destroying God's perfect creation after contaminating the food and water, he also destroyed the air we breathe.

Nick Begich, Jr., son of the late Alaska congressman of the same name, explains in *Why in the World are They Spraying?* that the U.S. Air Force has been using a technique called ionospheric heating to perturb the atmosphere for the past 30 years. It all began with a strange array of antennas erected in Begich's home state, called the High Frequency Active Auroral Research Program (HAARP). A high-energy radio frequency beam is generated by the array in order to heat part of the earth's ionosphere.

The general idea of high-intensity RF beams (or rays) was first proposed by the electrical genius Nikola Tesla in the early 20th century, and later patented by physicist Bernard Eastlund. According to the patent,

"Weather modification is possible by, for example, altering upper atmosphere wind patterns or altering solar absorption patterns by constructing one or more plumes of atmospheric particles which will act as a lens or focusing device." Even the course of the country's jet stream can be altered, according to Begich, who wrote the 1995 book *Angels Don't Play This HAARP*.

HAARP was run by the U.S. Air Force until 2015, when the University of Alaska Fairbanks took control of the facility. (https://chemtrailsafety.com/chemtrails_contrails.html)

The enemy of life contaminated the foods we eat, the water we drink, and the air we breathe. On purpose.

Then, there are our thoughts to corrupt. In Gad Saad's (2020) book, *The Parasitic Mind*, we see how Satan has mixed up Truth in a tangle of feelings and emotions,

I conducted a quick, and obviously informal analysis of university mottos. I found that there were one hundred twenty-eight matches for the word truth, forty-six matches for the word wisdom, sixty-one matches for the word science and zero matches for the words emotion or feeling. For example, Harvard's motto is Veritas (truth) and Yale's is Lux et veritas (light and truth). These venerable institutions of higher learning were not founded on an ethos of feeling but on the dogged pursuit of truth. And yet, across all our institutions from universities to the media to the social justice system to the political arena, truth is taking a back seat to feelings. This is true in the United States, it is true in Canada, and it is true across most of the western world" (p. 27).

Feelings are not facts. Satan would have us believe otherwise.

It is no small wonder our Lord and Savior Jesus told the woman at the well,

"Everyone who drinks of this water will be thirsty again; but whoever drinks of the water that I will give him shall never be thirsty; but the water that I will give him will become in him a fountain of water springing up to eternal life." (John 4:13-14)

And it is comforting to know Jesus said to them, "I am the bread of life; the one who comes to Me will not be hungry, and the one who believes in Me will never be thirsty" (John 6:35).

Next, we will discover just who these powerful people are today and from where they are waving their magic wands.

Chapter Twenty-Three
Who Is Holding the Magic Wand?

Follow the Money

And he led Him up and showed Him all the kingdoms of the world in a moment of time.
And the devil said to Him, "I will give You all this domain and its glory, for it has been handed over to me, and I give it to whomever I want. Therefore if You worship before me, it shall all be Yours."
Jesus replied to him, "It is written:
'YOU SHALL WORSHIP THE LORD YOUR GOD AND SERVE HIM ONLY.'"

Luke 4:5-8

Satan makes it obvious from his initial encounter with mankind in Genesis 3 that he has absolutely nothing but malicious intent for God's creation.

The Father of Lies is highly intelligent, despite being an arrogant fool. Satan knows if he approached God's people as a slimeball or a roaring lion he would be rejected by them, so he comes as an angel of light, as a flatterer, complete with a seductive smile. Without discernment, believers can be, and often are deceived. Satan presses relentlessly toward his goal, which is, of course, to lead people into destruction. Jesus says this about Satan in John 8:44,

> "He was a murderer from the beginning, and does not stand in the truth because there is no truth in him. Whenever he tells a lie, he speaks from his own nature, because he is a liar and the father of lies."

How can we tell if it's the enemy? When the Spirit of God is at work, all the glory goes to Jesus. When Satan is at work, the glory goes to the people he panders. Let's examine the world's monetary system to see how the enemy works promising power, control, and temporal riches using the world's currency.

Henry Kissinger, the former Secretary of State under President Richard Nixon, reportedly said, "Who controls the food supply controls the people; who controls the energy can control continents; who controls money can control the world."

Let's examine together who is regulating the world's money and who is controlling the world's wealth.

Several decades ago, I became aware of so-called "secret societies" who ruled the earth. I spent months researching the Skull and Crossbones as well as other fraternities from Yale University, the Illuminati and the Bilderberg Group. I've learned Freemasonry is the biggest, oldest, and most well-known secret society today. Each group exists in a powerful, unseen way. Working together, these groups manipulate the masses, tricking them into producing more wealth for the groups.

This is how Satan works in the dark, clandestine, and hidden from sight while actually in plain sight. The Mockingbird Media is complicit, all mainstream networks uncannily report the exact same lies day after day, believed by those without "ears to hear and eyes to see" (Matthew 13:16).

Many of those who control the CIA, the FBI, and many world agencies, operate under the guise of protecting people belonging to these underground networks of debauchery and greed. It will all surface. "For nothing is concealed that will not become evident, nor *anything* hidden that will not be known and come to light" (Luke 8:17).

So, who has secured the most wealth on earth?

> The Bible instructs us not to be ignorant of Satan's devices and it predicts that, as the Second Coming of Christ draws near, the world will be drawn into a One World Government, ultimately to be taken over by a Coming World Leader. The forces setting the stage for this final climactic chapter may have proceeded farther than most people realize.
>
> Few Americans know of the betrayal that was plotted on Jekyll Island, Georgia, which was destined to defraud Americans of their wealth and opportunity, and would eventually lead to the subjugation of our great democratic experiment to a centralized global dictatorship.
>
> In November of 1910, after having consulted with Rothschild banks in England, France, and Germany, Senator Nelson Aldrich boarded a private train in Hoboken, New Jersey. His destination was Jekyll Island, Georgia, and a private hunting club owned by J.P. Morgan.

Aboard the train were six other men: Benjamin Strong, President of Morgan's Bankers Trust Company; Charles Norton, President of Morgan's First National Bank of New York; Henry Davidson, senior partner of J. P. Morgan; Frank Vanderlip, President of Kuhn Loeb's National City Bank of New York; A. Piatt Andrew, Assistant Secretary of Treasury; and Paul Warburg. The secret meeting, as described by one its architects, Frank Vanderlip, went as follows:

> "There was an occasion near the close of 1910 when I was as secretive, indeed as furtive, as any conspirator. I do not feel it is any exaggeration to speak of our secret expedition to Jekyll Island as the occasion of the actual conception of what eventually became the Federal Reserve System." We were told to leave our last names behind us. We were told further that we should avoid dining together on the night of our departure. We were instructed to come one at a time... where Senator Aldrich's private car would be in readiness, attached to the rear end of the train for the South.
>
> Once aboard the private car, we began to observe the taboo that had been fixed on last names. Discovery, we knew, simply must not happen, or else all our time and effort would be wasted..."

The goal was to establish a private bank that would control the national currency. The challenge was to slip the scheme by the representatives of the American people. Earlier, it had been called the Aldrich Bill and received effective opposition. The devious planners of the revised bill titled it "The Federal Reserve Act" to mask its real nature. It would create a system controlled by private individuals who would control the nation's issue of money. Furthermore, the Federal Reserve Board,

composed of twelve districts and one director (The
Federal Reserve Chairman) would control the nation's
financial resources by controlling the money supply
and available credit, all by mortgaging the government
through borrowing."

(https://themillenniumreport.com/2017/12/the-
federal-reserve-system-its-not-federal-and-theres-no-
reserve/)

The Federal Reserve, despite what most Americans believe, is not
Federal and there is no reserve. The Federal Reserve is a completely
independent agency comprised of privately-owned banks.

Three years after President Woodrow Wilson signed the Federal
Reserve Act into law, Wilson made this astounding confession,

A great industrial nation is controlled by its system
of credit. Our system of credit is concentrated. The
growth of the Nation, therefore, and all our activities
are in the hands of a few men, we have come to be the
worst ruled, one of the most completely controlled
and dominated Governments in the civilized world
no longer a Government by free opinion, no longer a
Government by conviction and the vote of the majority,
but a Government by the opinion and duress of a small
group of dominant men.

A vast majority of Americans don't understand that
there is a connection between the Federal Reserve and
the federal income tax. The Revenue Act was enacted
in 1913, which was not a coincidence (Sanger, 2020,
p.368).

We are told to be "wise as serpents and gentle as doves" (Matthew
10:16). Satan has had his hands in our pockets since Eden. There
will come a day when we realize we've been duped by the devil. The
monies collected by the Federal Reserve fund projects for the special
interests of the wealthy, so they can become wealthier.

One example today can be found in the incredible amount of tax dollars being sent to the descendants of the Khazarians in modern day Ukraine. Their leaders claim to be Jewish; we already know what Jesus has to say about that in Revelation 3:9.

> To get an excellent overview of the world of international banking including the private banking cabal, and the Federal Reserve System, this interview, "The Gods of Money: How America was Hijacked," with F. William Engdahl is a must-listen. Engdahl is an award-winning geopolitical analyst, strategic risk consultant, author, professor and lecturer. Engdahl is the author of the trilogy, "Seeds of Destruction: The Hidden Agenda of Genetic Manipulation," "Myths, Lies, and Oil Wars" and "Gods of Money: Wall Street and the Death of the American Century." This 59 minute, revealing interview was conducted by Bonnie Faulkner on "Guns & Butter." "We Hold These Truths" has analyses and podcasts about the Federal Reserve System and its war financing mechanisms. (https://whtt.org/who-controls-the-money-controls-the-world/)

Additionally, *The Wealth Record* online offers this: A Jewish businessman, John D. Rockefeller was a well-known industrialist and philanthropist in America. He rose to fame as the founder of the Standard Oil Company, which dominated the oil industry. He became one of the wealthiest men at the age of 25. Rockefeller is regarded as one of America's leading businessmen and is known for helping to shape the U.S." (https://www.thewealthrecord.com/)

John D. Rockefeller's family was worth a staggering $340 Billion in 2022.

There is no truth, nothing good, no love, and no hope that can ever come from Satan. It's important to remember how when we allow the words of the enemy to have any power whatsoever in our lives, we willingly, by free will, come into agreement with things that directly oppose God's Word. Satan's desire is to "kill, steal, and destroy" anything that brings God glory, including bringing destruction to any person in his path.

The Rockefeller's massive wealth was used to shape our government and health care delivery system as we know it today.

Satan promises; he never delivers. He's a liar. He promises freedom and happiness but brings only slavery and sorrow. He promises power and new life, but conveys only weakness and death.

The Bible warns, "The way of the unfaithful leads to their destruction" (Proverbs 13:15).

Satan can and will control our very souls if we decide the corporal riches of this world are our god. Those who have chosen to worship Satan's money trick do not yet realize they've been duped.

Let's look at some more lies ...

Chapter Twenty-Four

Outer Space and Inner Turmoil

The Lie of Insignificance

And I heard every created thing which is in heaven,
or on the earth, or under the earth, or on the sea,
and all the things in them, saying,
"To Him who sits on the throne and to the Lamb be the blessing,
the honor, the glory, and the dominion forever and ever."

Revelation 5:13

The Canopy, the Light, the Dark, Food, Beauty, Creative Work, God's creation included everything we needed to survive, to thrive, and to be fulfilled. God created the perfect sky and a beautiful earth and He instilled in us the blessed feeling of satisfaction in doing creative work to sustain ourselves, thriving in His glory.

It's very simple, really. Either we believe what God says in the Holy Bible, or we don't. Either we have faith in His words, or we don't. Either we believe the Bible is divinely inspired, or we don't. There is no wiggle-room, there are no loopholes. It is written, "eternal life, which God, who cannot lie, promised long ages ago, but at the proper time manifested, even His word" (Titus 1:2-3).

> Satan likes to call God's integrity into question. But as we see in today's verse, it is impossible for God to lie— it's against His very nature. It's impossible for God to tell a lie, and it's nearly impossible for Satan to tell the truth. In the Garden of Eden, he pulled Eve away from God using a lie that sounded good to her.

> This is every Christian's battle. Satan starts by introducing a little lie and casting doubt. We believe the Bible is the Word of God because Jesus said it was the Word of God. If Jesus was wrong about that, then He was in error, which would mean he could not be the Son of God. We know Jesus could not be in error and be God as well. So the Bible is the Word of God.

> Satan wants us to doubt God's Word. Whether we'll admit it or not, we've all failed to act on His Word. We often turn to other sources of assistance in dealing with money, family, life, priorities, and choices.

> Ground your every decision in the Word of God, and Satan will not gain a foothold in your life. (https://tonyevans.org/blog/do-you-believe-gods-word)

Reading God's account of His creation, He tells us,

> In the beginning God created the heavens and the
> earth. And the earth was a formless and desolate
> emptiness, and darkness was over the surface of the
> deep, and the Spirit of God was hovering over the
> surface of the waters. Then God said, "Let there be an
> expanse in the midst of the waters, and let it separate
> the waters from the waters." God made the expanse,
> and separated the waters that were below the expanse
> from the waters that were above the expanse; and it was
> so. God called the expanse "heaven." (Genesis 1:1-2,
> 6-8)

Gratefully born again by the fullness of God's love and mercy, I
have been reading, studying, and living His Word only because of His
grace since the 1990s. I will admit, I didn't pay attention to God's
account of creation or the language of the firmament for a long time.
Asking His Holy Spirit to bring me the Truth, I began to read the
account of creation literally instead of figuratively. After all, we either
believe His Word, or we don't. I do, every single Word.

When delving deeper into information about the firmament, I
found it incredible, and prayed about it. Faith. I came to the point
of child-like faith in His Word. Faith that what God was telling us is
100% true.

Now, when I walk outside and look at the sky, I know it is blue
because of water, and it makes so much more sense. There literally
are waters above and below us on earth. I now see the earth as an
enclosed system. In the Garden of Eden, the firmament was secured,
creating a perfect greenhouse-like environment for humanity. After
the first temptation leading to the fall of mankind, the firmament,
although still in place, no longer was perfect. We know how during
the time of Noah, God opened the floodgates of heaven (the
firmament) to flood the earth, and opened the springs from below.

Space is the vast region of the firmament. Above the sky are waters which were already in existence before the earth was created. God sits above water. This is why Genesis 1 verse 2 says the "Spirit of God hovered over the waters before He created the earth."

If you are interested in seeing Biblical flat earth visuals, they are easily found in books and in videos when you search the Internet using the keywords, "Hebrew Flat Earth."

NASA is a mind-blowing satanic project. It has known the earth is flat for a long time. NASA research papers admit this fact:

> NASA Technical Memorandum 81238; *A Mathematical Model of the CH-53 Helicopter* (Page 17, Equations of Motion) *"The helicopter equations of motion are given in body axes with respect to a flat, nonrotating Earth."*
>
> (https://ntrs.nasa.gov/archive/nasa/casi.ntrs.nasa.gov/19810003557.pdf)
>
> (https://www.galileolied.com/post/15-nasa-research-papers-admit-flat-nonrotating)

Indeed, another example of how Satan works, putting everything out in the open for us to find, to believe or reject. His open display of deception is a complete mockery of God's precious gift to mankind of free will; too arrogant to think, too lazy to discern, too passive to question the truth, too smug to even wonder, most people blindly believing whatever they are told.

Here is another short video on www.Bitchute.com uncovering and proving the satanic roots of NASA: https://www.bitchute.com/video/dGsFNuetkP5o/.

More information about the shape of God's earth can be found by researching the CIA Operations Fishbowl, Highjump, Dominic, Blue Beam and Paperclip.

Using reverse ordinal gematria to calculate the value of the words, "National Aeronautics and Space Administration," you'll find the letters added together have a sum of "666." Finding it hard to believe?

Look at the derivatives:

Strong's Concordance
nasha: to beguile, deceive
Original Word: אָשַׁנ
Part of Speech: Verb
Transliteration: nasha
Phonetic Spelling: (naw-shaw')
Definition: to beguile, deceive
NAS Exhaustive Concordance
Word Origin
a prim. root
Definition
to beguile, deceive
NASB Translation
come deceitfully (1), deceive (8), deceived (3), deluded (1),
utterly deceived (1).

Source: NAS Exhaustive Concordance of the Bible with Hebrew-Aramaic and Greek Dictionaries. Copyright © 1981, 1998 by The Lockman Foundation

Why have we been duped into believing NASA is good? Why have we been conditioned to believe the earth is a globe spinning around a sun? The motive is two-fold. Simply follow the money. Billions of our taxpayer dollars have been used by NASA, the money flowing from the Federal Reserve. The photos of the vast universe are fake; they're photoshopped. There is not one single true photograph of the earth taken from "space."

Secondly, what better way for Satan to have us believe we are a speck of insignificance in a godless world? Satan presented mankind with a fake, vast universe where we are nothing more than a speck of nothingness, when, in truth, God knows "the number of hairs on each one of our heads" (Matthew 10:30).

Do you know the name of the founders of NASA? I'll tell you. Wernher von Braun, Lyndon B. Johnson, L. Ron Hubbard, and

Jack Parsons. Von Braun was a member of the Nazi SS, Johnson was the 36th president of the United States and was sworn into office following the November 1963 assassination of President John F. Kennedy, Hubbard was the founder of the Church of Scientology, and Parsons was involved in Thelema, the occultic religion founded by Aleister Crowley.

> Esmeralda Santiago once said, "Tell me who you walk with, I'll tell you who you are." Based on who was involved in NASAs creation, one has to wonder who or what NASA really is. If you are the company you keep, then NASA is an [*sic*] profane, occultic organization. That being said, what are the real motivations of NASA? Is it really all about rocketry and exploration or is there something more sinister going on behind the scenes?

> (https://vocal.media/futurism/nasa-s-dark-origins)

Remember, Jesus *ascended* into heaven (Acts 1:9-11) and He *descended* into Hades (Ephesians 4:9-10) to release innocent souls held in bondage. Jesus will come back in glory from the heavens, "BEHOLD, HE IS COMING WITH THE CLOUDS, and every eye will see Him, even those who pierced Him; and all the tribes of the earth will mourn over Him. So it is to be. Amen" (Revelation 1:7).

So, wonder with me. Why would Satan target space and the earth itself? The answer becomes obvious. Satan thrives on controversy and division. What topic would Satan want us all to argue about? Creation. God's Creation.

Fasten your seatbelt for the next big lie.

Chapter Twenty-Five
Modern Day Sorcerers

Selling Sickness for Power and Profit

And the light of a lamp will never shine in you again;
and the voice of the groom and bride will never be heard in you again;
for your merchants were the powerful people of the earth,
because all the nations were deceived by your witchcraft.

Rev 18:23

Billionaire John D. Rockefeller is often referred to as the father of modern medicine. He has an interesting, albeit dubious background.

[John's] father was a con artist and a bigamist. The tycoon's father, William Avery Rockefeller, was a traveling snake-oil salesman who posed as a deaf-mute peddler and hawked miracle drugs and herbal remedies. The smooth-talking huckster dubbed "Devil Bill" alternately fathered children, including the future industrialist, with his wife and mistress, the couple's live-in housekeeper. The itinerant William Rockefeller also lived a double life posing as an eye-and-ear specialist named Dr. William Levingston, and in 1855 he secretly married another woman.

Every year, [John] Rockefeller celebrated the anniversary of landing his first job. On September 26, 1855, a Cleveland merchant company, Hewitt and Tuttle, hired the teenaged Rockefeller as an assistant bookkeeper. From that year forward, the corporate tycoon celebrated "job day" every September 26 to commemorate his entrance into the business world, and he considered the date more important than his birthday. "All my future seemed to hinge on that day," he reminisced later in his life, "and I often tremble when I ask myself the question: 'What if I had not got the job?'"

Shortly after the discovery of petroleum in Titusville, Pennsylvania, the 24-year-old Rockefeller entered the fledgling oil business in 1863 by investing in a Cleveland refinery. In 1870, he formed the Standard Oil Company of Ohio along with his younger brother William, Henry Flagler and additional investors.

Through secret alliances with railroads, accumulating segments of the supply chain to achieve economies of scale, buying out and intimidating rivals and serving the growing demand for quality kerosene, Standard Oil eventually controlled 90 percent of the refining capacity of the United States. In the 1880s, Rockefeller moved Standard Oil's headquarters to New York City.

(https://www.history.com/news/10-things-you-may-not-know-about-john-d-rockefeller)

Rockefeller controlled almost 90% of America's oil. Soon, the possibility of creating everything from oil was discovered. Everything from solvents to skis to cortisone is produced from petroleum. He realized he could manufacture pharmaceutical drugs from petrochemicals derived from oil. Rockefeller's plan for the medical industry ran into one problem: the popularity of natural medicine in the United States.

Petrochemicals provide the chemical building blocks for most medicinal drugs: nearly 99% of pharmaceutical feedstocks and reagents are derived in some way from petrochemicals. For example, aspirin has been manufactured from benzene, produced in petroleum refining, since the late 19th century. (https://www.americangeosciences.org/geoscience-currents/non-fuel-products-oil-and-gas)

But Rockefeller's plan to use petrochemically-produced medicines faced a huge obstacle, and that was the favored use of natural medicines to treat illnesses.

In the 1930s, natural compounds were the primary substances dispensed for treating infections. Other poisons, such as turpentine and petrochemicals, were administered. However, any thorough study of pre-World War II pharmacy reveals the true nature of medicine in America. A review of old medicine bottles reveals that natural medicines were the mainstay, and this was the case throughout much of America for over 200 years. While certain early medicines were poisons or the so-called snake oils containing ingredients like kerosene, turpentine, arsenic and mercury, the majority were derived from various natural ingredients/herbs such as goldenseal, echinacea, ginger, Seneca, balsam, burdock, wintergreen, cinnamon and dozens of others. In fact, regarding the toxins it was often major business interests, including the early drug houses, which produced such chemical potions, including the House of Rockefeller. In fact, it was the latter, notably through John D. Rockefeller, which popularized the most noxious chemical drug of all: crude oil. (Ingram, 2016, pp.11-12)

It appears as though John. D. Rockefeller was walking in the footsteps of his snake-oil selling father, William Rockefeller, who posed as the fake doctor, Dr. William Levingston.

Pre-Rockefeller medicine, nearly all of the medical colleges and doctors in America were practicing holistic medicine, using extensive knowledge from Europe and Native American traditions. Herbal medicines were popular in America in the early 1900s.

Rockefeller knew in order to get control of the American medical system he would have to decimate the existing holistic community of practitioners who would be his competition.

His first move was to use his immense wealth from oil to purchase part of the German pharmaceutical company, I. G. Farbenindustrie AG, commonly known as IG Farben.

Controlling a drug manufacturing company allowed him to move forward with his plan to eliminate the competition.

It's important to note a few facts about IG Farben:

During World War II, IG Farben established a synthetic oil and rubber plant at Auschwitz in order to take advantage of slave labour [*sic*], the company also conducted drug experiments on live inmates. (https://www.britannica.com/topic/IG-Farben)

Several books shed light on the co-dependence of the military industrial complex that enabled the Third Reich to execute the Holocaust. I.G. Farben – Hell's Cartel – was THE pivotal company without whom Hitler could not have implemented his industrialized "scientific" Holocaust. "IG (Interessengemeinschaft) stands for 'Association of Common Interests': The IG Farben cartel included BASF, Bayer, Hoechst, and other German chemical and pharmaceutical companies. As documents show, IG Farben was intimately involved with the human experimental atrocities committed by Mengele at Auschwitz. A German watchdog organization, the GBG Network, maintains copious documents and tracks Bayer Pharmaceutical activities."

(https://ahrp.org/auschwitz60-year-anniversary-the-role-of-ig-farben-bayer/)

Existing medical specialties pre-Rockefeller included chiropractic, naturopathy, homeopathy, holistic medicine and herbal medicine. Rockefeller hired a contractor named Abraham Flexner to eliminate the competition by submitting a report to Congress in 1910.

The report deviously "concluded" that there were too many doctors and medical schools in America. The report also accused natural healing modalities, which had existed for hundreds of years, of being unscientific quackery. The report called for the elimination of the quackery, and the standardization of medical education. The report established the AMA (American Medical Association, another monopoly) which would grant medical school licensure in the U.S.

Although Flexner's report had some valid points, the motive for the report was completely driven by Rockefeller's compulsion to have complete control of the medical system. Based on that report,

Congress pursued Flexner's recommendations, enacting new laws directly related to how medical practitioners would practice. The 1910 Flexner Report established the foundations of our modern medical system, labeled "Rockefeller medicine."

> With new laws in place, Rockefeller teamed up with Andrew Carnegie and started funding medical schools all over America on the strict condition that they only taught allopathic medicine. Through the power of their huge "grants", this powerful team systematically dismantled the previous curricula of these medical schools, removing any mention of the healing power of herbs or natural treatments. Teachings on diet and other natural (non-drug) treatments were also completely removed from medical programs.
>
> After removing traditional medicine from medical schools, Rockefeller made sure to secure his monopoly by launching a targeted smear campaign against his competitors. Homeopathy and natural medicines were discredited and demonized through the newspapers and other media of the time. Some doctors were even jailed for using natural medicine treatments, including treatments that had been used safely and effectively for decades before.
>
> One shocking fact that I found while researching this post was that Rockefeller didn't stop at U.S. borders. He actually went into China to spread Western Medicine. To quickly summarize what happened in China: The China Medical Board (CMB) was created in 1914 by the Rockefeller Foundation (RF) and provided with a $12 million grant. The RF's goal was to "modernize medical education and to improve the practice of medicine in China". They started by building a hospital in Beijing (Peking Union Medical College, opened in 1919), but they were unable to

expand to other locations (as planned) due to mounting expenses.

In short, the diligent work of Rockefeller and Carnegie was a smashing "success". They crushed the underfunded, grassroots competition and created our current medical system. This system continues today wherein "Big Pharma" makes large "donations" to medical schools in exchange for teaching the medical students to use their patented drugs. As part of this system, many alternative treatments are criminalized. For example, by law, it is illegal to treat cancer with any modality except chemotherapy, surgery or radiation. It is actually a criminal felony for a medical practitioner to treat cancer with anything but these three modalities. Why is this the case? Follow the money. The average cost of cancer treatment is $150,000, so clearly Rockefeller and his precedents were keen to keep the monopoly on this one. And of course, the American Cancer Society was founded by none other than John D. Rockefeller in 1913.

(https://meridianhealthclinic.com/how-rockefeller-created-the-business-of-western-medicine/)

After the Flexner Report, the AMA only endorsed schools with a drug-based curriculum. It didn't take long before non-allopathic schools fell by the wayside due to lack of funding. (https://www.thelibertybeacon.com/john-d-rockefeller-used-ama-take-western-medicine/)

Rockefeller then used the AMA, condoning widespread use and endorsement of petrol-based drugs, toxic vaccines, chemotherapy and radiation, to destroy the competition which it eventually did do by regulating medical schools. Sickness became a business to sell for profit and power.

John D. Rockefeller became the nation's first pharmacist, peddling magical pills to fix any problem. A greedy, lying snake-oil salesman, just like his father. The AMA was established to treat illnesses with pharmaceuticals, eradicating the use of natural, holistic remedies for healing given to us by our Creator.

Revelation 18:23

And the light of a candle shall shine no more at all in thee; and the voice of the bridegroom and of the bride shall be heard no more at all in thee: for thy merchants were the great men of the earth; for by thy sorceries ("sorceries" Greek Word 5331 *Strong's Exhaustive Concordance*)

ALL NATIONS DECEIVED.

"Sorceries"
G5331 (Strong)
φαρμακεία
pharmakeia

From G5332; medication
("pharmacy"), that is, (by extension) magic (literal or figurative): -
sorcery,
witchcraft.

Chapter Twenty-Six
For Thee and Not for Me

Magic and Medicinal Murder

Woe to those who call evil good and good evil,
who put darkness for light and light for darkness,
who put bitter for sweet and sweet for bitter!
Isaiah 5:20

Your mind believes everything you tell it.

 You will believe what your teachers tell you because, well, they know. Right? They are teaching you what they have been taught. You believe your physician when he/she tells you your diagnosis and tells you the best treatment plan, right? They are following the protocol they've learned in medical school, right?

After all, your mind will believe everything you tell it.

What if your teachers were lied to and they believed it? That means you have learned a lie they accidentally told you. What if your doctor was getting you hooked on pills because that's the protocol he learned, and he believes it's the best treatment available? What if doctors knew those pills were going to do more harm than good? Would they still prescribe them if their license may be at risk if they don't? How would you know?

Isn't this how magic works?

> Magic allows you to experience the impossible. It creates a conflict between the things you think can happen and the things that you experience. While some magicians would like you to believe that they possess real magical powers, the true secret behind magic lies in clever psychological techniques that exploit limitations in the way our brains work. Many of these limitations are very counterintuitive which is why we can experience the magical wonder of the impossible."
>
> (https://theconversation.com/tricking-the-brain-how-magic-works-56451)

Magic causes cognitive dissonance.

> The theory of cognitive dissonance proposes that people are averse to inconsistencies within their

own minds. It offers one explanation for why people sometimes make an effort to adjust their thinking when their own thoughts, words, or behaviors seem to clash with each other.

There are a variety of ways people are thought to resolve the sense of dissonance when cognitions don't seem to fit together. They may include denying or compartmentalizing unwelcome thoughts, seeking to explain away a thought that doesn't comport with others, or changing what one believes or one's behavior.

(https://www.psychologytoday.com/us/basics/cognitive-dissonance)

In other words, a truth may be unbearable or just plain too uncomfortable to process, much less accept, so one will lie to themselves about it or completely dismiss it in order to feel comfortable again.

Satan really likes this trick a lot.

This is precisely why God tells us in Proverbs 28:26, "One who trusts in his own heart is a fool, but one who walks wisely will flee to safety." And, of course, it's also why He told us in Proverbs 9:10, "The fear of the LORD is the beginning of wisdom, And the knowledge of the Holy One is understanding."

Nowadays, the Western World doesn't look for the actual cause of a medical problem, rather, the Rockefeller model, melded within the legal framework of our nation, tells us only the symptoms are treated with medicines. This seriously lacks logical thinking, because it means everybody who has the same symptom set or even seems to have the same symptom set will receive the same treatment. This is called the Medical Protocol, brought to us by the American Medical Association (AMA). Here's the legal definition:

Medical protocol means any diagnosis-specific or problem oriented written statement of standard procedure, or algorithm, promulgated by the Medical

Director as the medically appropriate standard of out-of-hospital care for a given clinical condition.

(https://www.lawinsider.com/dictionary/medical-protocol)

So, in a supposedly free country, I can't make an independent decision regarding a personally preferred course of treatment, because a medical professional has already decided for me which treatment I need. If I go against or dare to challenge the given medical protocol, I risk being dismissed by the practitioner, which of course gets charted in the main data bank.

Modern medical magic brought to us by sorcerers and thieves!

Just look at how far we've fallen from God's intents and purposes for us, His beloved creation. We have drifted away from Him, we have forgotten about His gifts to us and His healing power, we have pushed aside His precious gift of free will to decide what is holiest and best for our health and well-being. We have forgotten we are "temples of His Holy Spirit" (1 Cor 6:19).

What better way for Satan to interfere with God's creation than to confuse children about gender? American Academy of Pediatrics (AAP) has new guidelines supporting gender change for children. The American Academy of Pediatrics is an organization of 67,000 pediatricians committed to the optimal physical, mental, and social health and well-being for all infants, children, adolescents, and young adults.

In September of 2018, the AAP urged parents to accept the preferred gender identity of their children without regard for the children's actual biological sex.

Now, the Academy is urging parents to approve of "surgical intervention" and puberty-blocking hormones for what they've labeled as, "gender-confused youth."

"The transition-affirming movement purports to help children," American College of Pediatricians (ACPeds) president Dr. Michelle Cretella has said. "However, it is inflicting a grave injustice on them and their non-dysphoric peers."

Medical professionals have been advocating this uncontrolled experimentation using the myth that people are born transgender. "There is no rigorous science that demonstrates gender identity is inborn and unchangeable," Cretella told LifeSiteNews. "There is no rigorous science that establishes all gender identities are equally healthy and fixed for all children and teens. There is a long history of scientific literature to indicate that the vast majority of young children with gender dysphoria outgrow it by late adolescence," she added.

(https://www.lifesitenews.com/news/american-academy-of-pediatrics-new-guidelines-support-gender-change-for-kid/)

In April of 2021,

The American Medical Association (AMA) today urged governors to oppose state legislation that would prohibit medically necessary gender transition-related care for minor patients, calling such efforts "a dangerous intrusion into the practice of medicine." In a letter to the National Governors Association (NGA), the AMA cited evidence that trans and non-binary gender identities are normal variations of human identity and expression, and that forgoing gender-affirming care can have tragic health consequences, both mental and physical.

(https://www.ama-assn.org/press-center/press-releases/ama-states-stop-interfering-health-care-transgender-children)

According to Cleveland Clinic's website:

Common transgender surgery options include:

Facial reconstructive surgery to make facial features more masculine or feminine.

Chest or "Top" surgery to remove breast tissue for a more masculine appearance or enhance breast size and shape for a more feminine appearance.

Genital or "Bottom" surgery to transform and reconstruct the genitalia. (https://my.clevelandclinic. org/health/treatments/21526-gender-affirmation-confirmation-or-sex-reassignment-surgery)

Of course, anyone who does not go along with these new protocols, this satanic agenda which permanently disfigures children, is labeled "intolerant."

The Epoch Times reported this in August of 2022, in an article titled, "Teachers Who Do Not Affirm Gender Identities Accused of Harming Children":

Do you remember when you first heard of the terms "nonbinary" or "gender fluid"? How about "gender-expansive" or "gender-nonconforming"? I bet it was within the past five years.

I recently came across a guide distributed to teachers and administrators nationwide. The guide was made in partnership with the American Civil Liberties Union, the National Education Association (the largest teachers union in the United States), and LGBT groups. The guide is titled "Schools in Transition: A Guide for Supporting Transgender Students in K–12 Schools." So what's in this nationally distributed guide?

It states: "The expression of transgender identity, or any other form of gender-expansive behavior, is a healthy, appropriate and typical aspect of human development. A gender-expansive student should never be asked, encouraged or required to affirm a gender identity or to express their gender in a manner that is not consistent with their self-identification or expression. Any such attempts or requests are unethical and will likely cause significant emotional harm."

It continues: "Ongoing learning is a key element of this process. Educators and administrators need to engage in regular professional development and training to build a school climate that avoids gender stereotyping and affirms the gender of all children. (https://www.theepochtimes.com/teachers-who-dont-affirm-gender-identities-accused-of-harming-students_4691405.html)

Futuristic author George Orwell predicted,

> Nearly all children nowadays were horrible. What was worst of all was that by means of such organizations as the Spies they were systematically turned into ungovernable little savages, and yet this produced in them no tendency whatever to rebel against the disciple of the Party. On the contrary, they adored the Party and everything connected with it. All their ferocity was turned outwards, against the enemies of the State, against foreigners, traitors, saboteurs, thought-criminals. It was almost normal for people over thirty to be frightened of their own children. (Orwell, 1949, p. 24)

We are just about there. Do they not see this is just one more way of "thinning the herd," of killing off humanity? The modern-day sorcerers, cutting on these children, skewing their young minds, murdering their identities with medicine, will have a huge problem in the end with their latest trick on God's creation. "But whoever causes one of these little ones who believe in me to sin, it would be better for him to have a great millstone fastened around his neck and to be drowned in the depth of the sea" (Matthew 18:6).

The Satanists, thinking we are all under their demonic spell, think they have succeeded in creating a new reality.

Chapter Twenty-Seven
Who Do You Think You Are?

The Manipulators of Madness

God created us, giving us the precious gift of free will. His Holy Spirit helps us to discern right from wrong, goodness from evil.

How many Americans even believe in God?

> Most recently, Gallup found 81% of Americans expressing belief when asked the simple question, "Do you believe in God?" This was down from 87% in 2017 and a record low for this question first asked in 1944, when 96% believed. It reached a high of 98% in the 1950s and 1960s.
>
> (https://news.gallup.com/poll/268205/americans-believe-god.aspx)

Let's look at the birthrate in this country:

> The U.S. birthrate has fallen by 20% since 2007, with no signs of reversing. This decline cannot be explained by demographic, economic, or policy changes.
>
> (https://econofact.org/the-mystery-of-the-declining-u-s-birth-rate)

How does this nation view the sanctity of life?

> According to the Guttmacher Institute's Abortion Provider Census, a total of 930,160 abortions were carried out in the U.S. in 2020, an 8% rise from 2017, when the last report was published. Around one in every five (20.6%) pregnancies ended in abortion in 2020, up from 18.4% in 2017, the census found.
>
> (https://www.forbes.com/sites/siladityaray/2022/06/15/abortion-rates-in-the-us-rose-in-2020-after-30-years-of-decline-report-says/?sh=3e8d00486985)

The total number of abortions in the U.S. between the years of 1973-2020? 63.6 million +. (https://www.all.org/abortion/abortion-statistics).

And yes, you read that correctly: "Around one in every five (20.6%) pregnancies ended in abortion in 2020, up from 18.4% in 2017." (https://www.forbes.com/sites/siladityaray/2022/06/15/abortion-rates-in-the-us-rose-in-2020-after-30-years-of-decline-report-says/?sh=3e8d00486985)

These statistics clearly represent a nation in deep moral decline. Remember, Satan cannot create life, so in his jealousy of God and his rage toward Him, he will do everything to destroy life, clone it, even replace it:

> I had watched a Timpool IRL livestream a little back where he said that there is some kind of artificial intelligence using Humans to bring itself into existence and I also hear from all Christians who say with the state of the current world that it is the end times and everyday it looks more and more like the Day of Judgment in the Bible.
>
> I find it interesting these two things seem to be happening at the same time and this coming from me a non-Christian. The fact that something from the Bible that was talked about for thousands of years in scripture is unfolding before our eyes and Artificial Intelligence is coming into existence before our eyes from what I keep seeing from companies like Facebook, Twitter, Amazon and other Big Tech companies making in terms of A.I. advancement to track us. I wonder if artificial intelligence will be ... Satan?
>
> The Bible speaks about Satan coming into existence on our Earth during the end times and could artificial intelligence be that incarnation that Satan takes as a foothold in our world. Think about [*sic*] A.I. is being marketed to us the unsuspecting consumer as

something that will give us anything we desire and all we have to give up to it is our privacy.

Satan in the Bible is said to make bargains with random people giving them anything they want that they desire for their immortal soul. Artificial Intelligence will give you anything you want to buy from Amazon or Ebay which is like Satan giving people whatever they want and in return, you give up your privacy which is like your soul both you can't get back once you give them away.

Artificial Intelligence wants to destroy Humanity and so does Satan ... is not out of the realm of possibility that Satan and artificial intelligence are one in the same?

Artificial Intelligence will reach everywhere in our lives when it fully comes online from what we buy on Amazon to what we say on Facebook, that sounds like Satan having power over everyone and everything. Just something to think about people. ¯ Blood Ranger

(https://www.geeksandgamers.com/topic/could-artificial-intelligence-be-satan/)

Think. Take a deep breath. Pray with me for eyes to see and ears to hear (Matthew 13:16).

The ethical questions surrounding AI have long been the subject of science fiction, but today they are quickly becoming real-world concerns. Human intelligence has a direct relationship to human empathy. If this sensitivity doesn't translate into artificial intelligence the consequences could be dire. We must examine how humans learn in order to build an ethical education process for AI.

AI is not merely programmed, it is trained like a human. If AI doesn't learn the right lessons, ethical problems will inevitably arise. We've already seen examples, such as the tendency of facial recognition software to misidentify people of colour [*sic*] as criminals.

(https://ethics.org.au/injecting-artificial-intelligence-with-human-empathy/)

Released in 2002, Spielberg's *Minority Report* showcased breakthroughs in CGI (Computer Generated Imagery). The film focuses on a policeman, played by Tom Cruise, trying to prove his innocence in a corrupt, dystopian world where law enforcement can arrest people before they commit a crime.

[Cruise] is the head of a sensational new development in law-enforcement, being tested out in Washington DC by a private security corporation. Cruise is in charge of "pre-crime", catching murderers before they commit the deed: a technique which harnesses the prophetic powers of three "pre-cogs" mute visionaries dreaming and drifting in a flotation tank, heads connected up to software which projects their presentiments on to a giant screen. Cruise then manipulates and enlarges these with the grandiloquent cybergloved hand gestures of a hi-tech Toscanini or histrionic traffic cop, looking for clues as to where to send in his SWAT team...

More pertinently, it is just about possible to read *Minority Report* as a brilliant allegory for a hi-tech police state which bullies villains and law-abiding citizens alike with self-fulfilling prophecies of wrongdoing: a new kind of thoughtcrime, intentioncrime, perhaps.

(https://www.theguardian.com/film/2002/jun/28/culture.reviews)

Twenty years later, today:

> In the United States, a piece of software called
> Correctional Offender Management Profiling for
> Alternative Sanctions (Compas) was used to assess
> the risk of defendants reoffending and had an impact
> on their sentencing. Compas was found to be twice as
> likely to misclassify non-white defendants as higher risk
> offenders, while white defendants were misclassified as
> lower risk much more often than non-white defendants.
> This is a training issue. If AI is predominantly trained
> in Caucasian faces, it will disadvantage minorities.
>
> (https://ethics.org.au/injecting-artificial-intelligence-
> with-human-empathy/)

The world appears to be in the death throes of Satan:

> Pure evil, going so far as to implement transhumanism.
> While most people understand transhumanism to
> be the blending together of machine and the human
> body, when you begin to understand the foundations of
> Artificial Intelligence and Quantum Computing, you
> realize that this is even more sinister.
>
> People have had nanotechnology injected into their
> bodies. They're called the covid-19 vaccines. I mean,
> that's what they are. We know through the blood work
> that people are having metals show up in their body;
> copper, tin, aluminum ...
>
> Looking at artificial intelligence, and nobody was
> warning us about biotechnology, about gene editing
> technology, and these scientists play God. But that's
> what happened. These scientists were playing God
> in biotech and scientists were playing God in AI. So
> in biotech, they were making their own species by
> deleting, copying, and pasting and creating new multi-
> species beings.

They have humanized pigs and things like that. It's disgusting what they've created. Then with AI, they're creating these humanized cyborgs that have human tissue because they've converged with biotech ...

These mad scientists are moving beyond the physical realm of simply human bodies and technology, and actually incorporating the spiritual, or demonic, as well. When you think about it, if this is true then this is the return of Genesis 6 and the Nephilim, literally using AI as the Trojan horse to create human/demon hybrids.

(https://freedomfirstnetwork.com/2022/09/ artificial-intelligence-is-being-injected-into-humans- is-this-the-return-of-the-genesis-6-nephilim)

Yuval Noah Harari is from Kiryat Ata, Israel. He is one of three children born to Shlomo and Pnina Harari. They are a secular Jewish family with roots in Lebanon and Eastern Europe. Yuval is a member of the World Economic Forum (WEF) and is a top advisor to its founder Klaus Schwab.

Harari provided insight into the mindset of what is commonly referred to as "the global elite" during an economics summit in 2020. At this summit Harari warned that humans were, "no longer mysterious souls, but rather hackable animals." Harari also stated at the summit, "Biological knowledge multiplied by computing power multiplied by data equals the ability to hack humans." (https://sociable.co/military-technology/yuval-harari-hackable- humans-wef-darpa-preconscious-brain-signals/)

Spiritual slovenliness combined with intellectual laziness is a dangerous combination. People have sidled up to their television sets since the 1950s, slowly slipping into a state of stupor. The masses have been brainwashed for so long, all manners of evidence can be presented, simply to be dismissed by the dazed as dis-information.

Think about it, television is "Telling a Vision" complete with "programs" for programming.

Mark Twain said, "It's easier to fool people than to convince them they've been fooled."

What if, just what if, wonder with me, what if a way could be developed to inject humans with nanotechnology, targeting areas of the brain to deaden the brain's hippocampus, short-circuiting neural pathways to erase thoughts, perceptions, memories while obliterating emotional response?

Indeed, human intelligence has a direct relationship with human empathy. Care. Compassion. If empathy cannot be duplicated since it is as much a gift from our Creator as free will, then the enemy will have to find a way to destroy it.

Introducing the new Brain Report tentatively scheduled to be implemented in 2025:

> *Brain Research Through Advancing Innovative Neurotechnologies* (BRAIN) Working Group Report to the Advisory Committee to the Director, NIH. View BRAIN 2025 Report (PDF, 1254KB).
>
> The human brain is the source of our thoughts, emotions, perceptions, actions, and memories; it confers on us the abilities that make us human, while simultaneously making each of us unique. Over recent years, neuroscience has advanced to the level that we can envision a comprehensive understanding of the brain in action, spanning molecules, cells, circuits, systems, and behavior. This vision, in turn, inspired The BRAIN Initiative®. On April 2, 2013, President Obama launched The BRAIN Initiative® to "accelerate the development and application of new technologies that will enable researchers to produce dynamic pictures of the brain that show how individual brain cells and complex neural circuits interact at the speed of thought.

(https://braininitiative.nih.gov/strategic-planning/
brain-2025-report)

After all, one must first find out how individual brain cells and complex neural circuits work before one can either find a way to use them or obliterate them altogether.

In 2021, "An Overview of Micro Nano Swarms for Biomedical Applications" was published by Hui Chen, Huimin Zhang, Tiantian Xu, and Jiangfan Yu. Each of the researchers share the Shenzhen Institute of Artificial Intelligence and Robotics for Society (AIRS) in Shenzhen in common.

The Abstract states, in partial:

> This review presents the recent progress of micronanoswarms [*sic*], aiming for biomedical applications. The recent advances on structural design of artificial, living, and hybrid micro nano swarms are summarized, and the biomedical applications that could be tackled using micro nano swarms [*sic*] are introduced, such as targeted drug delivery, hyperthermia, imaging and sensing, and thrombolysis. Moreover, potential challenges and promising trends of future developments are discussed. It is envisioned that the future success of these promising tools will have a significant impact on clinical treatment.
>
> (https://pubs.acs.org/doi/10.1021/
> acsnano.1c07363)

Since Artificial Intelligence cannot duplicate the language of the heart, manipulators will attempt to make it "useless."

Do not believe them.

They want to own us. They want to literally change our minds. They want us to give our souls to them.

Chapter Twenty-Eight
Life on the Pharm Forever

Mockery of Free Will

We have been duped. Beguiled. Deceived.

> It is astounding that just one lie can neutralize the
> majority of Christians. That's right. Neutralize.
> This lie takes us out of the game and turns us into
> mere spectators in the epic story of Christianity that
> continues to unfold in every generation. This one lie
> is largely, if not primarily, responsible for ushering in
> the post-Christian modern era throughout Western
> civilization. It may be the devil's greatest triumph in
> modern history. This is the holocaust of Christian
> spirituality.
>
> In a thousand ways every day we tell ourselves and
> each other that holiness is not possible. We don't
> use that language, but the fact that the word *holiness*
> has disappeared from our dialogue is proof that we
> consider it either irrelevant or unattainable. When was
> the last time you heard someone speak about holiness.
> (Kelly, 2018, p.33)

Recall the global health crisis which began in 2020. It was called a pandemic, causing fear and panic world-wide. At the same time, please recall the Rockefeller model of medicine founded on the pharmacological foundation of prescribing drugs to treat illnesses as opposed to using natural healing techniques.

Now, after nearly three years, the truth about the COVID mRNA shot/vaccine, implemented for emergency use to abate and abolish COVID-19, is being told.

Does the mRNA "vaccine" alter human DNA? There are two opposing answers:

> SPIKEVAX (elastomeren) is the second mRNA
> vaccine to receive provisional approval in Australia.

mRNA vaccines use a synthetic genetic code called RNA to give our cells instructions about how to make the coronavirus' unique spike protein. When our body has made the protein encoded by the mRNA vaccine, it then recognizes the spike protein as being foreign and launches an immune response against it. The RNA from the vaccine does not change, or interact, with our DNA in any way.

(https://www.tga.gov.au/news/news/covid-19-vaccine-spikevax-elasomeran)

The other scientific opinion is this:

Two of the COVID-19 vaccines available in the US use messenger RNA technology to prevent or reduce the symptoms of COVID-19 infection. This mRNA vaccine technology is new; the consequences of altered DNA, if any, are unknown.

Other scientists believe that mRNA vaccines can enter and permanently alter DNA. Like DNA vaccines, RNA vaccines use part of the genetic code of the virus to get the immune system to respond.

(https://www.medicaldaily.com/can-mra-vaccine-change-dna-459011)

So, does it affect human DNA? You decide. Free will. Go to the Throne of our Creator and ask Him.

This is what the developer of the mRNA shot says about it:

Dr. Robert Malone, the key developer of the mRNA technology in the Pfizer-BioNTech and Moderna vaccines, said the findings were "buried" in the study, which was published by the journal *Cell*. He described the results as a potential "health public policy nightmare."

Unlike typical vaccines, which use a live virus that has been attenuated, or weakened, the messenger RNA vaccines carry genetic material that instruct cells how to produce the spike protein, which activates the body's immune response and produces antibodies.

Malone said that having worked with mRNA for decades, he found the persistence of the synthetic spike protein in lymph node germinal centers to be "highly unusual."

The study quantitatively measured spike protein levels in plasma after vaccination. And it turned out that the levels are higher than the levels observed in a person with a severe COVID-19 infection.

Malone wrote that "the fact that this (is) [*sic*] only now being discovered, or if it was known, released to the public is criminal in my opinion. (https://www.wndnewscenter.org/health-nightmare-dr-robert-malone-spotlights-study-on-mrna-spike-protein/)

Prominent cardiologist Dr. Peter McCullough, an epidemiologist, has this to say about the mRNA shot:

It's known that the vaccines have a "dangerous mechanism of action," which is "the production of the spike protein."

"The spike protein is what makes the respiratory infection lethal, and it follows that in some people excessive production of the spike protein in a vulnerable person would be lethal after a vaccine," he said.

McCullough has found from his review of studies that the lipid nanoparticles which deliver the spike protein in the mRNA system "go right into the heart." He believes that's why studies indicate a higher-than-expected rate of myocarditis, particularly in boys, associated with the vaccines. And the studies show that the myocarditis produced by a COVID-19 infection tends to be mild and "inconsequential" while the myocarditis caused by the vaccine can be severe.

"When the kids get myocarditis after the vaccine, 90% have to be hospitalized," McCullough said in a podcast interview in December [2021]. "They have dramatic EKG changes, chest pain, early heart failure, they need echocardiograms." (https://www.wndnewscenter.org/health-nightmare-dr-robert-malone-spotlights-study-on-mrna-spike-protein/)

Both doctors have been de-platformed and discredited on social media sites and have been publicly chastised by the mainstream media. Doctors, researchers, and anyone who attempted to speak out about the dangers of the mRNA shot or alternative treatments for anyone who supposedly has gotten COVID-19 have also been silenced by the mainstream news sources, banned from social media platforms, and punished by the AMA.

David Martin, Ph.D. is one of the persons brave enough to talk about it anyway.

Dr. David Martin is the founder and owner of the company M-CAM International which has provided research and corporate advisory services to over 160 countries and he has personally served as an advisor to the World Bank and many governments. Dr Martin first came to the attention of the world when he [was] featured in the August 2020 documentary by Mikki Willis called Plandemic Indoctornation.

Dave wrote his first classified briefing about bioweapons corruption in 2001, and has been presenting lectures at bio-weapons conferences since then. He has been tracking Dr. Anthony Fauci's spending and notes that Fauci has authorised [*sic*]

$191 billion in funds for the bio-weaponisation [*sic*] of viruses against humanity. (https://totalityofevidence. com/dr-david-martin/)

Dr. Martin has introduced evidence that SARS-CoV-2 is a manmade bioweapon, and has been in the works for decades. He discovered this man-made bio weapon was funded by the National Institutes of Allergy and Infectious Diseases (NIAID) under the direction of Dr. Anthony Fauci.

Martin has been in the business of tracking patent applications and approvals since 1998. His company, M-Cam International Innovation Risk Management, is the world's largest underwriter of intangible assets used in finance in 168 countries. M-Cam has also monitored biological and chemical weapons treaty violations on behalf of the U.S. government, following the anthrax scare in September 2001.

According to Martin, there are more than 4,000 patents relating to the SARS coronavirus. His company has also done a comprehensive review of the financing of research involving the manipulation of coronaviruses that gave rise to SARS as a subclade of the beta coronavirus family.

In his testimony to ACU, he reviews some of the most pertinent patents, showing SARS-CoV-2 is not a novel coronavirus at all but, rather, a manmade virus that has been in the works for decades.

Up until 1999, coronavirus patents were all in the veterinary sciences. The first coronavirus vaccine to use the S spike protein was patented by Pfizer in January 2000 (Patent No. 6372224). It was a spike protein virus vaccine for canine coronavirus. You can look up the actual patents for yourself on the United States Patent and Trademark Office's website.

(https://www.citizensjournal.us/patents-prove-sars-cov-2-is-a-manufactured-virus/)

And then there is this:

> Dr. Ryan Cole is a Mayo Clinic trained, board-certified anatomic pathologist, clinical pathologist, as well as he studied immunology and virology. At the America's Frontline Doctors White Coat Summit, Dr. Cole revealed what the Mockingbird media, corrupt drug pimps in DC and Big Pharma do not want you to know. It's amazing to watch the self-appointed, bought-and-paid-for, useful idiot fact-checkers fall all over themselves to cover for Big Pharma and their deadly poisons, but they do it in spite. Recently, they have gone after my personal page in an attempt to claim false information and out of context nonsense. However, they will not address what is killing the people who take these shots. In fact, you will NEVER see them write what is actually killing these people who took the shot and were dead within minutes to a few months. They go along with the narrative of "COVID," which has never been proven to exist in the first place and not one doctor, nurse, employee of the CDC, the FDA or any other government around the world can supply a single COVID isolate. Yet, this scientist shows exactly what takes place in the body of someone who has died and what the autopsy reveals.
>
> (https://www.citizensjournal.us/want-to-see-the-effects-of-the-covid-shots-in-autopsies-this-scientist-shows-you-video/)

Dr. Malone adds: "Individuals who have received multiple COVID booster shots are increasingly the ones being hospitalized, and in some cases dying, because of what Dr. Robert Malone describes as 'immune imprinting.'" (https://www.worldtribune.

com/dr-malone-highly-vaccinated-suffering-worse-outcomes-than-those-with-natural-immunity/)

As of June 1, 2022, "More than 11.8 billion doses of coronavirus vaccines have been administered, in at least 197 countries worldwide," with 61% of the world fully vaccinated. (https://www.bbc.com/news/world-56237778)

> The more you look into Big Pharma and so-called medical "science," the more you realize it's all a massive, coordinated, greed-driven fraud to sell prescription medications to people who don't need them and won't be helped by them.
>
> Essentially, Big Pharma and the complicit pharma-funded corporate media have been committing massive medical fraud for decades, lying to the public and promising that SSRI pills will make you happier. In reality, it only made Big Pharma richer. The entire industry is rooted in fraud and fake science. (https://www.naturalnews.com/2022-07-29-vast-majority-of-pharmacology-science-published-research-is-a-complete-fraud.html)

Why would doctors and hospitals offer an emergency-use-only medicine without clear outcomes being known?

The answer is sinister. Demonic, really. It's all about power and money. Satan's tools. Lies, Deception. Population control. The Internet of Bodies. The linking of human AI machines.

Did these doctors know? Were they and were the hospitals complicit? The answer is buried online under an avalanche of cover-ups. You still can find out how much COVID-19 relief money the health care providers in your state received here: https://www.statnews.com/2021/09/24/covid-19-relief-money-providers-in-your-state/

The global population is projected to reach 8 billion on 15 November 2022 according to the United Nations website:

https://www.un.org/en/desa/world-population-reach-8-billion-15-november-2022

The Abstract for the article, "Culling the Herd: Eugenics and the Conservation Movement in the United States, 1900-1940" explains it in these chilling words:

> While from a late twentieth- and early twenty-first century perspective, the ideologies of eugenics (controlled reproduction to eliminate the genetically unfit and promote the reproduction of the genetically fit) and environmental conservation and preservation, may seem incompatible, they were promoted simultaneously by a number of figures in the progressive era in the decades between 1900 and 1950. Common to the two movements were the desire to preserve the "best" in both the germ plasm of the human population and natural environments (including not only natural resources, but also undisturbed nature preserves such as state and national parks and forests). In both cases advocates sought to use the latest advances in science to bolster and promote their plans, which in good progressive style, involved governmental planning and social control."
>
> (https://pubmed.ncbi.nlm.nih.gov/22411125/)

Face it.

It's the silent "shot," heard only in whispers of fear, seen only in the lifted arms ready and willing to receive its needle, its treachery manifested in the maimed and murdered in the years ahead.

Chapter Twenty-Nine

Forgive Us!

Fooled and Fouled

Be of sober spirit, be on the alert.
Your adversary, the devil, prowls around like a roaring lion,
seeking someone to devour.

1 Peter 5:8

The LORD said to Satan, "Where have you come from?" (Job 2:2).

"Well I've been patrolling the earth, I've been looking around my estate." And he had. Now let's get this clear, that doesn't mean that God is helpless in this world. It does mean and we've got to think this through, that God is allowing Satan to be prince of this world and god of this world. He's allowed it. And people say, "What does God think He's doing allowing that?" Well, I would just say my only answer to that one is, what's He doing allowing you to be like you are? Why should you blame Him for allowing Satan to rebel when He allowed you to?

The answer is very simple. He's a Father and He will not force any of His creatures to go His way and He gives you freedom to rebel. And we can't grumble about His giving the angels freedom, though they have superior intelligence and strength because He gave us the same freedom and we've used it in the wrong way.

Genesis describes his devices, and Revelation describes his doom, and he hates those two books. And there have been more scholarly attacks on the book of Genesis than any other book and more attempt to turn it into myth and legend and away from fact than any other book in the Bible. Why? Because Satan doesn't want you to believe Genesis 3 ever happened. He doesn't want you to know how he got hold of Eve. He doesn't want you to believe that he said what he did to that first married couple, and he attacks the book of Genesis.

But the other book which he hates more than any other is the book of Revelation, because as you read through that book, you come to a point where it says that the devil himself will be cast into the lake of fire, Revelation 20:10. Do you know that Jesus told us to pray every day about the devil? Matthew 6:9-13, the original prayer that he taught His disciples when they said Lord, teach us to pray. He said pray like this: Dad in heaven, then pray for the things He wants, His name, His will, His Kingdom, then He said pray for the things you need, you need food, you need forgiveness, and then He said finish by praying this, "deliver us from the evil one." We've turned evil into a thing in our thinking. It's not a thing, it's a person. There's no evil anywhere in the universe apart from persons. Evil is an intensely personal thing. There's no love in the universe apart from persons who love. And so, evil is personal. And Jesus said pray daily, deliver us from the evil one. Start your prayer by thinking of your Dad in heaven, but end your prayer by thinking of the devil on earth and go out to face him."

(https://www.facebook.com/3n1Ministry/videos/722475555567045)

Just look at what Satan has done! Ask yourself, "What have I allowed him to do in my life? What has he done to my family?" Weep. Fall to your knees and pray. Ask for forgiveness. Beg for mercy. The days will get shorter, God's love is forever.

Our Creator gave us everything we needed to survive and to thrive. He gave us perfect health, a perfect environment to sustain us with delicious foods to nourish our bodies. Our Father gave us perfect pleasure found in imaginative work, discovered in His plan for creation.

We've listened to the evil one tickling our ears with better pleasures, more of this, more of that, and we listened! We believed the father of lies, the devil of deception!

We refused to believe there were demons, we laughed in the face of temptation. We've ruined our lives, and the lives of others, and we've scoffed at the very existence of our Savior.

Lord, JESUS, God Almighty, forgive us!

He sent his Holy Spirit to help us, to comfort us, to console us, and what did we do? We ignored Him. We thought we could do it all by ourselves. We made messes of our lives and blamed Him for our own decisions.

We believed in magic. We believed the lie.

> The most compelling evidence that magic, witchcraft and sorcery still exist and are practiced both openly at lower levels, and secretly at high-powered levels can be found in the book of Revelation. In 9:21, we find the world in a war where 33.3 percent of the world's population is killed. Notice that despite all this devastation where some 2 or 3 billion people (or more) will be exterminated, those rebels who influence world affairs in covert ways, and those in a less threatening manner, still practice magic arts. In 18:23, we read that the same virgin of Babylon spoken of earlier has controlled world governments and commercial activity by magic spells. This is not some metaphor or symbol. Those who call on Satan to influence world affairs use magic and sorcery just as Christians use prayer and faith to ask for the Lord's help! Remember, Satan wants to copycat the Eternal Father. Still do not believe? Read 21:8 and 22:15. Those who practice magic arts do not have any place in the kingdom of God and will be burned in the fiery lake of burning sulfur, the second death. The temptations of Jesus Christ also gives us clues into sorcery and magic. In Matt. 4:3, Satan, the father of sorcery, witchcraft and magic, tries to seduce Jesus into practicing a form of alchemy by turning bread into stones. In verse 6, he tries to

get Jesus to practice a form of magic called levitation, where one's body is suspended in mid-air. Then finally, Satan puts on the biggest seduction of all. In verse 9, he offers Jesus the whole world, including control over the affairs of men. Of course, Jesus never intended to succumb to Satan's temptations. So why did He want these temptations to be recorded? Because He wanted us to see how Satan has tempted all the chosen leaders of the Eternal Father's people (both racially and spiritually) throughout history. Many of them, even today, have given in to these temptations which is why the whole world is deceived.

(https://believersweb.org/the-truth-about-magic-witchcraft-and-sorcery/)

We stopped paying attention, taking everything for granted. We got fat. We got sick. We got sick of everything except ourselves.

The medical gurus made us sicker, shoving medicines down our throats and shooting us up with poisons on purpose. Did they know? How could they not have known? It was their job to "do no harm."

Was all medicine suddenly evil? Of course not. That is how the father of lies works, though. The champion of confusion throws in a truth here, an antidote there, so we lazily end up believing the whole bushel of lies.

Many Christians wrestle with their decisions over accepting valid medical therapies, including the use of prescription drugs. The Bible does not give us much on this subject, but if we examine the purposes of prescription drugs we can present an ideal approach to their uses based on biblical principles. We know from Scripture that ill health, disease, and death are the result of sin in the world. Much of Jesus' earthly ministry involved combatting that curse, as He healed people everywhere He went (see Matthew 15:31).

Jesus is the exact representation of God's being (Hebrews 1:3), and by healing people He showed us God's compassion and His identity as the Great Physician who will one day restore all of creation to health (Romans 8:18–22).

So, it is clear from Jesus' ministry that to seek healing is not wrong; in fact, it is very right! Also, Luke, the writer of both the Gospel of Luke and Acts, was a physician (Colossians 4:14). Dr. Luke may not have dispensed prescriptions in the manner that doctors do today, but he was in the business of treating people's physical ailments, using the medicines and treatments of his day.

In the days before prescription drugs, people sought relief from pain in other ways. Alcohol is mentioned in Proverbs 31:6–7 as being given to the terminally ill and others who suffer. Also, in 1 Timothy 5:23, Paul advises Timothy to drink a little wine to relieve his stomach ailment. Since other drugs had not yet been developed, fermented drinks were often used as remedies for pain and suffering, and the use of such analgesics is approved in God's Word.

Also, we should keep in mind that most of today's prescription medicines are based on elements occurring naturally in creation. A doctor may prescribe Amoxil, for example, but where did that antibiotic come from? It came from a substance produced by a blue-green mold called Penicillium notatum. Where did the mold come from? God made it. So, we can say that God created the penicillin mold and gave it the useful property of killing infectious bacteria. God then allowed people to discover this property, isolate the acting agent, and purify it for use in the human body. Is it wrong to use God's own creation to improve the health of humanity? Not at all. In fact, He is glorified in such discoveries. Yes, and the children of God must never allow themselves to be brought under the habitual control of a substance (see 1 Corinthians 6:12 for this principle stated in a different context).

In the end, a Christian's use of prescription drugs is between that Christian and the Lord. The Bible does not command the use of medicinal treatments, but it certainly does not forbid it, either. The child of God should care for his or her body as being the temple of the Holy Spirit (1 Corinthians 3:16). This means taking preventative care, maintaining a healthy diet, and getting proper exercise. It also means taking advantage of the wisdom that God has given skilled researchers and physicians. We understand that God is the Healer, no matter by what means He heals, and we give the glory to Him. (https://www.gotquestions.org/Christian-prescription-drugs.html

Nonetheless, so-called Christians ran to get in line to get shot up, without going to His Holy Throne to ask Him what to do first. How many times did our Father tell us not to be afraid? Hundreds of times. Yet, there they were, knees knocking in fright, rolling up their sleeves to be maimed and murdered by the Satanists.

Jesus wept (John 11:35). His Father will spread His holy wrath over the earth (Revelation 16:1).

This is Satan's last hurrah, and he knows it. He's working hard to corrupt our DNA. Why? Because we are created in the image and likeness of our Creator. Satan seeks to destroy our ability to love, to care. He seeks to enslave us, making us nothing more than walking AI machinery. "And in those days people will seek death and will not find it; they will long to die, and death will flee from them!" (Revelation 9:6).

Satan is blurring our sexuality, making a mockery of God's pro-creative act creating new life. Men are dressing like women,

women like men. Pharmacies hand out hormones like candy on the instructions of the doctors.

Satan whispers into the ears of fornicators to kill their inconvenient babies, calling the child a blob of cells, not yet human. Moloch, the ancient demon god who feeds on human sacrifices, celebrates the death of these children. The organization called Planned Parenthood gladly chops up the dead baby's body, selling the child's parts to the highest bidder.

> The video is gruesome and appalling. It purportedly shows a Planned Parenthood executive sipping a glass of wine in a Los Angeles restaurant while casually explaining how they sell body parts from aborted babies.
>
> The undercover video was filmed in July 2014 by the Center for Medical Progress, an advocacy group that reports on medical ethics. They dispatched two actors posing as representatives of a human biologics company to a business lunch with Deborah Nucatola, Planned Parenthood's senior director of medical services.
>
> (https://www.foxnews.com/opinion/shock-video-planned-parenthood-sells-dead-baby-body-parts)

Satan's hatred toward God burns in darkness forever (John 3:20), never satisfied. He prowls the earth, finding new victims to feed to his pal Moloch.

The disasters caused by the shot started surfacing in the Spring of 2022:

> But the biggest house of lies that is falling apart is the one surrounding these shots they have spent more than a year trying to convince us are safe and effective vaccines and spent the same amount of time trying to force us all to take ... but thanks to some unknown hero, we now have internal documents prepared by

Pfizer, expos[ing] the whole truth about the adverse health events suffered by the people who participated in their vaccine trial.

We have the information. And here's what it tells us. It tells us about more than twelve hundred fatal adverse events from people who received the Pfizer shot, out of 42,000 reported adverse events.

This document has a nine-page list of "adverse events of special interest." Just to pick out a few at random: Acoustic neuritis, aortic embolus, Cerebellar embolism, Crohn's disease, epileptic psychosis, infantile spasms, meningitis, swollen tongue.

(https://www.redvoicemedia.com/2022/03/top-secret-pfizer-documents-leaked-pfizer-knew-that-vaxx-would-kill-thousands/)

They knew. They serve Satan.

Chapter Thirty
God Reigns Forever

Trust Him

Jesus responded and said to him, "Truly, truly, I say to you, unless someone is born again he cannot see the kingdom of God." Nicodemus said to Him, "

How can a person be born when he is old?

He cannot enter his mother's womb a second time and be born, can he?"

Jesus answered,

"Truly, truly, I say to you, unless someone is born of water and the Spirit, he cannot enter the kingdom of God."

(John 3:3-5)

Jesus lived, taught, rose from death, and sent His Holy Spirit to us. God does not dwell in buildings built by human hands, rather, He dwells in each one of us who have been born again in His Spirit. Our Savior lives through His people, His church. "Do you not know that your body is a temple of the Holy Spirit within you, whom you have from God, and that you are not your own?" (1 Cor 6:19).

The world seems to be crumbling. Trust Him. He is with us. "The kings of the earth take their stand and the rulers conspire together against the LORD and against His Anointed, saying, 'Let's tear their shackles apart and throw their ropes away from us!'" (Psalm 2:2-3).

The blood of Jesus saved us, so it stands to reason Satan would target our bloodstream. "For the life of the flesh is in the blood" (Leviticus 17:11). Satan sees victory over God by attacking our flesh by tainting and/or poisoning our blood.

> "COVID spelled backwards is DIVOC. *Divoc* in Hebrew means 'Possession of the evil spirit.' Sorcery is a derivative of the Greek word 'Pharmakeia' and this is the word from which we get the word 'Pharmacy.' Sorcery also implies 'Witchcraft.' They're luring your soul with their spells and rituals to break the connection between you and your spirit (GOD) because they know that you're the TRUE TEMPLE OF GOD."

> In the Bible, *pharmakeia* carried with it the idea of sorcery, occultism, and black magic. It is in this sense that Paul used the term in Galatians 5:20 as the word "witchcraft."

> Back then, apothecaries were your go-to for drugs and medicines. but did you know they also specialized in potion-making? And we know just how abominable

potions really are, as they correlate and tie right in to magic, sorcery, and witchcraft.

(https://safeguardyoursoul.com/pharmakeia-and-sorcery/)

"And the light of a lamp will never shine in you again; and the voice of the groom and bride will never be heard in you again; for your merchants were the powerful people of the earth, because all the nations were deceived by your witchcraft" Revelation 18:23.

If the evil ones had their way, the earth would be filled with minion worker-slaves to use for their own benefit. Humans would be reduced to an AI transhuman existence, owning nothing, existing in a META universe of make-believe, serving Satan and his followers, as the intertwined, Internet of Bodies.

God knows our struggles. We are called to stay faithful to Him, just as Job stayed faithful to Him.

You see, Satan, the ultimate deceiver, knows this is not about battling flesh and blood rather, it is against the spiritual forces of evilness. He does not want us to know, though, gleefully torturing us in the process.

Armor up! (Ephesians 6:10-18)

Never forget Satan knows the Bible word for word. He uses it against us.

Fr. Michael Hinton, biblical scholar, co-author of the book *Flipping Tables*, and cherished friend, reminds us of this truth:

> For 500 years we have had the Bible in the language of the people, which is the greatest accomplishment of the Reformation. Yet, it is shocking, even among so-called reformed people, how many hold on to man-made doctrines that contradict Scripture.
>
> Ignorance is no excuse for anyone who can read.
>
> Two possible explanations are carnality and demonic activity. The money-grubbing churches preach easy

anti-gospels to please people, who reward them with more money. The devil asked from the beginning, planting a thought in the head, "Did God say ...?"

So are revealed the enemies of mankind: the world (money), the flesh (easy, man-made doctrines), and the devil (questioning and rejecting the clear Word of God in Scripture).

People are waking up, continuing to pray, delving into God's Word. "See that no one deceives you with empty words, for because of these things the wrath of God comes upon the sons of disobedience" (Ephesians 5:6).

The Luciferians slowly are being exposed. The "fake" Jews are falling.

> The takedown of the Khazarian mafia is accelerating. A worldwide arrest warrant issued for David Rockefeller Jr. means one of their top bosses is now a hunted man. Meanwhile, riots and demonstrations around the Western world are bringing down other KM leaders like Emmanuelle Macron of France and Justin Castro of Canada. Already, the Rothschild clan has admitted defeat and is now under the leadership of Nathaniel Rothschild. He promises that from now on his clan will stick to business and stay out of geopolitics. Here is a link to his company Volex. https://www.volex.com/
>
> (https://thegoodlylawfulsociety.org/worldwide-arrest-warrant-for-david-rockefeller-jr-as-khazarian-mafia-take-down-continues-by-benjamin-fulford/)

"God knows the outcome even when we can't see it. Having faith that God is good and faithful means trusting Him in every situation; continuing to pray and maintain hope even when it seems impossible or hopeless." (Nelson, 2020, p. 74)

What we are seeing in the world is Satan's agenda being played out. The Luciferians are serving their god, and we must separate ourselves from this world and serve our God. Satan is mighty, our God is Almighty.

When the going gets rough, I find myself being strengthened by the promise in Romans 8:28, "And we know that God causes all things to work together for good to those who love God, to those who are called according to His purpose."

This life-changing moment comes to mind:

> Mid-afternoon sunlight streaming through the stained-glass windows, I was practically alone in the little perpetual adoration chapel. There were a handful of ancient sisters sitting quietly in the surrounding pews. It was quiet and peaceful and I began my silent prayer.
>
> Dear Jesus Lord, keep my children safe, unbreak their hearts, heal them, heal me ... please ... please
>
> I nodded off, at least I thought I did. When I opened my eyes, I was sitting at a table at an outdoor cafe, a huge umbrella covering the whole table shielding it from the hot summer sun. I looked up and saw I was having lunch with Jesus. I sat up straight, looking down to make sure I was decently buttoned up.
>
> A beggar approached our table. He was unkempt and dirty, bones protruding through his very soiled tattered garment. I reached to give him some food from my plate.
>
> Jesus commanded, "No, don't do that!"
>
> Startled, I looked up and said to Jesus, "but he's hungry! Didn't You tell us to feed the hungry, give drink to the thirsty, clothe the naked, visit the imprisoned?" ... I rattled off the corporal works of mercy straight from the Book of Matthew describing His own words from His Sermon on the Mount. Then, I realized I was arguing with our Lord and Master Jesus Himself! I was embarrassed and stopped talking. I felt my face blush.

Jesus said softly, "Do not give him anything."

Totally confused, I asked Him, "I don't understand. Why not?"

Jesus said, "Because that's Satan. If you give him even the smallest piece of anything, he will keep coming back for more and more *until there is nothing left of you.*"

I was trying to do the right thing, the holy thing, following His holy directions and I realized I had it all wrong! Thoughts swirled. I was caught off-guard, out of context, in a different dimension.

I looked up at Him and asked, "How do I know when to give and who to give it to?"

"Trust Me," was His answer.

Immediately, I was delivered wide awake back to the wooden pew. I searched the chapel and thought loudly: Wait! Wait! Don't go! Where are you?

I realized, at that moment, I had no idea how to trust Him.

I had no idea what it meant to trust Him. During my life, I had prayed, I performed the works of mercy, I had taught my children how to pray, I had gone to church religiously and yet here I was, completely baffled.

I also realized at that moment, even though I thought I had trusted Him, I truly wasn't trusting Him at all and I had no idea what this really meant or how to do it. Oh, I had been kidding myself, the reality was clear: I had no idea. I looked around, searched for Him, silently in my heart pleading for Him to return to tell me how to trust Him! I needed to know.

My "lunch" with Him that day changed my outlook. I realize now I was not alone during the long years I spent searching for Him to give me the answer. He was answering me with every breath I took, with every step I was taking moving toward Him. I truly think everyone goes through a time like I did, wanting to know if He's real, searching for answers.

It's that ubiquitous "why" reverberating in our souls, our spirits, the universe, begging an answer. The spiritual desert is not a land of punishment; truly, it's a place of discovery, refreshment, refinement of the soul. (Nelson, 2020, pp. 74-76)

"No temptation has overtaken you except something common to mankind; and God is faithful, so He will not allow you to be tempted beyond what you are able, but with the temptation will provide the way of escape also, so that you will be able to endure it" (1 Corinthians 10:13).

And do not be conformed to this world,
but be transformed by the renewing of your mind,
so that you may prove what the will of God is,
that which is good and acceptable and perfect.

Romans 12:2

– End of Part Three –

God created a perfect world for us.

Gifted with free will, we decide whether we believe Him or not.

The evil one has worked hard to convince people God's Truth is a fairytale.

Indeed, God allowed Satan time to rule over the earth (1 John 5:19),

confident that those who love Him would do what He'd asked of them.

Satan knows his rule is limited.

Temporary. Ephemeral. Ticking away.

Frantically, he uses magic. Spells. Deception.

He wants to steal your soul.

He lies. He is the father of lies.

He will do anything. He's desperately hateful in his jealousy.

He is jealous of the Creator of life because he cannot create life!

So, he steals it.

Satan scoffs and mocks God,

as more and more of His children fall into sin.

He uses magic to create madness and mayhem.

We were warned the evil one would use medicine to fool everyone.

Revelation 18:23

And so he did.

The Battle is real. It's a spiritual battle.

We have been called to participate in His Glory

by telling everyone the end of the story!

God's HOLY SPIRIT is with us in these final days.

Believe Him!

EPILOGUE

*And we know that God causes all things to work together for good
to those who love God,*
* to those who are called according to His purpose.*

Romans 8:28

We think we're exempt, but we're not. We think we are weathered souls and our hearts can't break anymore, but they do.

Tell the Truth, they say. No opinions. Truth. The whole Truth and nothing but the Truth.

We used to lay a hand on a Bible, the only real Truth, to prove our intentions are honorable and good, our words Truthful.

I wonder how many people who were swearing by the Truth in that book even knew what was in it?

Satan knows God's Word, the Bible, forwards and backwards. He knows it better than any person on earth. He uses the words in it against us, skewing them, telling us it's alright to do this and that or some other sin, convincing us there's a loophole when there really isn't one.

So, amazingly, we often choose to believe him. We sin. We fall from grace and find ourselves at the edge of despair, void of hope, loveless, angry. Miserable.

~~~

My husband and I met with a married couple for lunch not long ago. Drizzly and grey, the weather matched the moods. Our friend was on the brink of filing for divorce; I had attended their wedding nearly forty years ago.

Over a decade ago, her husband decided he was a woman.

We'd met with them for dinner a few weeks earlier, so we already had experienced the strangeness of seeing her husband wearing a dress and heels. Years of hormone treatments were not going to remove his Adam's apple, or make his hands any smaller. No amount of feminine gesturing was going to detract from his broad shoulders and small hips. The pink sweater, the mascara, and the hair clip keeping the puff of bouffant in place were not going to soften the angular jawline or the long, narrow nose. He was trying hard, though.

His wife and I were good friends many years ago. We had recently resumed our friendship after I called her following a nudging in my heart around Christmas-time. Our friendship had been put on hold for decades while we lived our lives in different parts of the world, were busy raising our children, and just plain living life. It was nice to see her again.

She shared with me what happened, admitting to me how deeply she had suffered during her husband's transformation. It had been only recently that he finally admitted to her he had never considered what it would do to her, to their marriage. Stunningly, they had never discussed it. One day, he decided he was a woman and that was that.

Apparently, he hadn't noticed the torrent of tears she had shed during his transition process, or any of the frustration she felt. She admitted to me how she continued to feel abandoned and lonely from the lack of marital intimacy with her husband since that day.

She had stopped calling her "him" years ago, her brain either deadened from the pain, or reconditioned by societal norms to accept his new sexual identity. Rejected and deserted, she nonetheless continued to sleep together with "her" in their marital bed.

It had never occurred to him she had lost her husband, her intimate partner, his sturdy manly presence in her life. As far as he could see, he simply was doing what made him happy, and expected her to be happy for him. He kept his feelings front and center.

During the process, there was an incident when she became physically ill after finding a stash of slutty women's clothing and boots in bags in their basement. Then, she found wrappers from estrogen treatments in his coat pocket. He was not just cross-dressing. He was chemically altering himself.

The cognitive dissonance ate through her heart, poisoning her body. She fought a bout of cancer, her body sick from the confusion and anger that never abated.

She realized the only way for her to survive was to forge a unique friendship with this "new" person. She had lost her job and was too weak to look for another. He had lost his job, too, after boldly going to work dressed like a woman. Of course, they made a different excuse to fire him/her, the end result was the same, no employment.

Oh, she had convinced herself she was happy with the arrangement for years, stuffing her own thoughts deep inside her mind, her feelings never reaching her heart. She repeatedly emphasized how her husband was "still a person" who had feelings, and she was constantly aware of the need to not hurt "him/her," no matter what.

Their platonic friendship was a weird alliance. They went to the gym together, using the same women's locker room. His/her genitals had been shrunken from years of hormone treatment, and he/she wore special underwear to compress whatever was left under his/her swimsuit.

They ate meals together, went to movies together, pretending everything was alright. And it was, really, as long as his/her feelings were not hurt.

After years of this charade, my friend decided to end the marriage. She told him of her decision on a deep, dark day in December, describing she no longer could live a lie because she was not a lesbian and had no intention of becoming one. I wondered if this was the day God nudged me to call her after decades of silence.

He/she said he was saddened she wanted to divorce because he/she thought they could "beat the odds."

After all, he/she was happy. How could something so right turn out to be so wrong?

~~~

I looked out the window at the restaurant and saw my friend parking her car. Her husband was with her. I had wondered if (s)he would decide to stay home at the last minute. I watched them get out of the car and walk toward the restaurant.

I greeted him by his feminine name. My friend asked me to do this so he wouldn't be upset, cautioning me he would leave if I called him by his former masculine name. I felt like I was walking on eggshells. It didn't matter to them, as long as he/she was happy. As we walked to the table, I told him/her it was good to see them. He snottily said, "I'll bet" under his breath. I braced myself. He clearly was being combative.

Divorce is never easy, no matter what the circumstances. My heart was breaking for both of them. Their marriage was over and had been for a long time.

When I went to their wedding many years ago, a part of the religious ceremony beckoned the congregation to agree to support the marriage, to be there for them if they encountered any trouble. I agreed, of course. I reminded them of this and they nodded their heads in the affirmative, remembering. Taking a deep breath, I recalled for them that marriage is between a man and a woman, and how the marriage contract had been broken when he decided to become a woman.

My hope was to alleviate the pain and stress of the broken contract, with love and friendship staying intact. I wondered how he could continue to think his gender-change would not distort everything?

Stating this Truth set him off, and he started to shake, his voice quivering while he indignantly said, "That is not true. Here, in this nation, men can marry men and women can marry women!"

I responded, "You are speaking of secular marriages, not spiritual ones. I saw a spiritual union between the two of you decades ago. Marriage is between a man and a woman."

He literally was shaking, his scorn spilling all over the conversation. He hissed, "You hide behind your interpretation of the Bible. What you are saying does not apply to today. Let he who is innocent cast the first stone!" He shot a bitter look at me, got up from his chair, slammed his fists on the table, and said, "God is love!" Then, he stormed away from the table.

I asked my friend's permission to look for him. She shrugged her shoulders. I got up from the table to look for him.

Lost sheep. Maligned souls. God tells us to look for them and tell them about Him.

So, I did.

Her husband was nowhere to be found. I returned to the table. My friend got up from the table to look for him.

Returning to the table, she said she had found him outside the restaurant under a tree, crying. Her demeanor was different. She was visibly angry. She lashed out at me and accused me of making her husband cry.

A few weeks later, I received a scathing text message from her. I am now so hated in their household that they will not say my name out loud, she wrote.

They do not see their own dysfunction, their own problems, preferring to shift the focus onto someone else to blame for the mess they've created.

I called my Pastor. We prayed together. My husband and I were saddened by the whole situation. My Pastor said flatly, "They didn't want to hear the Truth, and they're keeping each other sick."

I know their hatred toward me is misdirected. Sin does this, I know it well. I used to do it, too. It's so much easier to blame someone else, taking the focus off of yourself. "The devil made me do it. It's not my fault. There's nothing wrong with what I am doing. You are not being loving enough." Excuses abound. The fact remains, it is about not wanting to hear the Truth. God's Truth.

Following His Gospel is hard. I know. You will lose friends. You lose family (Luke 21:16).

God wants all of His children to know His love and His mercy, without ever forgetting He is a just God, too. Our Father is a loving Father who does not put up with shenanigans.

So, I search for the fence-sitters, the spiritually blind and deaf, to tell them the Truth. How could I not? I am thankful for the people who awakened me from my own impending demise decades ago.

I recalled how my friend had told me, a few weeks earlier, how her husband had been trying to find a part in the Bible that said trans-gendering is allowed. It's not there.

He/she had asked her about being baptized in God's Holy Spirit. I truly had hoped He was ready to change, to realize what he was doing, to see the pain he had caused, the damage he had done to his family.

It was clear he/she wanted God's Word to change, he/she wanted validation for his/her decision, and as it turned out, so did his wife.

~~~

God knows the map of each person's heart. It's up to us to avail ourselves to Him, to be His hands and His feet until He returns in Glory.

False gospels have taken their toll. Satan is busier than ever breaking up families, confusing gender, attacking friendships, and corrupting children if he can't prevent them from being born in the first place.

God is love. This is absolutely true. What else is He, though? Apparently, my friend's husband had heard that part of the Gospel so many times he believed that was the end of it. It's not, though.

A few days earlier, this couple's daughter had nastily told them what she believed was a Biblical truth. My friend insisted she stop screaming and swearing at her, reminding her she was to honor her parents. Her daughter insolently replied, "Don't quote the Bible at me. Let he who is innocent cast the first stone. You have no right to tell me anything about the Bible."

Cherry-picking verses and quoting Scripture out of context without knowing the whole lesson has become commonplace in our broken world. True, Jesus said, "Let he who is innocent cast the first stone" (John 8:7). What is the rest of the story in that parable, though? Jesus, our Christ, told the woman in that story to "Go forth and sin no more" (John 8:11).

We are all sinners in need of a Savior. Accepting Jesus as our Lord and Savior changes everything. We strive daily to be more like Him, less sinful, as perfect in Him as we possibly can be.

Yes, God is love. What else is in the depth and breadth of God, though? God is a just God, He is our Creator, He is our Father. His ways are not our ways and we cannot even begin to understand Him. "For My thoughts are not your thoughts, nor are your ways My ways," declares the LORD" (Isaiah 55:8).

These scenarios are happening over and over in our dangerously corrupt world we are living in today. Daughters rising up against their mothers, families shattered by what the false gospels are telling us are acceptable sins of this age. Sin is encouraged to be accepted under the banner of, "God is love" therefore He loves us no matter what we do.

He loves us, yes. He created us. We are His children. We break His heart, though, every time we choose to disobey Him.

It's true. God does not send anyone to hell, we send ourselves there by the decisions we make. Free will. We get to decide.

His love and redeeming grace are our only hope, our salvation.

Indeed, Satan has been allowed to rule this earth. He prowls in search of souls to corrupt and steal. Our bad decisions, our sins, will crush us if we let him have his way.

People have come to believe the lie that we are the pride and joy of our Creator no matter what we do. This is one of the most prevalent and one of the deadliest of the false gospels.

Is the abortionist our Creator's pride and joy? Is the slanderer or fornicator His pride and joy? Is the murderer His pride and joy? Is the drag queen, who is reading to little children at the library, His pride and joy?

Of course not.

But realize this, that in the last days difficult times will come.

For people will be lovers of self, lovers of money, boastful, arrogant, slanderers,

disobedient to parents, ungrateful, unholy, unloving, irreconcilable,

malicious gossips, without self-control, brutal, haters of good,

treacherous, reckless, conceited, lovers of pleasure rather than lovers of God,

holding to a form of godliness although they have denied its power;

avoid such people as these.

For among them are those who slip into households

and captivate weak women weighed down with sins,

led on by various impulses, always learning,

and never able to come to the knowledge of the truth...

Now you followed my teaching, conduct, purpose, faith,

patience, love, perseverance, persecutions, and sufferings,

such as happened to me at Antioch, at Iconium, and at Lystra;

what persecutions I endured, and out of them all the Lord rescued me!

Indeed, all who want to live in a godly way in Christ Jesus will be persecuted.

But evil people and impostors will proceed from bad to worse,

deceiving and being deceived.

You, however, continue in the things you have learned and become convinced of,

knowing from whom you have learned them,

and that from childhood you have known the sacred writings

which are able to give you the wisdom that leads to salvation

through faith which is in Christ Jesus.

All Scripture is inspired by God and beneficial for teaching,
for rebuke, for correction, for training in righteousness;
so that the man or woman of God may be fully capable,
equipped for every good work.
(2 Timothy 3:1-7, 10-17)

For the love of God, and the salvation of your soul, believe Him.

Trust Him.

Disappearing into a vapor of dust

Annihilated
Along with the scoffers and thieves of dreams.

Broken promises, earthly delights
Gone in an instant.

Was it worth it?

Rattled, the serpent's tail swept the shattered lives
into the Inferno to be with him forever.

Under the earth,
The same earth where Satan had promised them sovereignty.

Instead, now trod upon by the faithful,
Utterly defeated.

They wail and gnash their teeth,
unseen under the holy feet above them.

Stepped on. Crushed. Confused.

The Victorious Ruler, the merciful, yet just Creator,
God Himself,
Sees all from His Throne.

Oh, they can hear the whispers of relief,
The shouts of joy;
The praise and thanksgiving

Above them.
Never ending.

Their evil plans, dissolved by the poisoned tears
of trickery.

Where did the magic go?

It never really existed.
The war had been won long before the first sleight of hand,
Satan knew it all along.

He lied.

GOD is

The great "I AM"

The Alpha and the Omega, the Conqueror of all evil,

Yesterday, today and forever.

A Few Words

It has taken me nearly 70 years to write this book.
I've had to live this long to be able to wonder so deeply,
love so fully,
Unwrap this gift of faith so providently,

believe so unwaveringly.

My heart has been broken over and over,
and I know now, only God's grace can glue it back together.

Indeed, God is writing this book,
He writes all of our books when we are His,
using our fingers to put it on paper
all glory to Him!

It's true. I am nothing without Him.

The rhythm of my breathing is from His breath of Life,
the tempo of my heart pulses me toward Him for eternity.
Please God, find me worthy.

Make my feet like the tips of matchsticks as I skate the edge of
Your Word
sparking the flame of Your Glory.

Make me worthy, Lord God.
Use me for Your Glory!
Heal us, open our eyes and our ears, and
deliver us all from the evil one.

Appendix A

The Strong Man and His Fruits

Or, how can anyone enter the strong man's house and carry off his property, unless he first ties up the strong man? And then he will plunder his house.

The one who is not with Me is against Me; and the one who does not gather with Me scatters.

Matthew 12:29, 30

Strongman	Fruit	Scripture Support
Spirit of Divination Attempt to foretell the unknown by occult, witchcraft.	Fortune-teller, rebellion, drugs, magic, hypnotist, horoscopes.	Micah 5:12, Isaiah 2:6, Isaiah 47:18, Exodus 22:18.
Familiar Spirit One who inquires of the dead, ability to contact the spirits passing them from generation to the next within receptive families.	Medium, yoga, drugs, clairvoyant, false prophecy, superstitions.	1 Chronicles 10:13, 1 Samuel 28, Isaiah 47:13, Exodus 22:18
Spirit of Jealousy Envy, malicious competition.	Envy, revenge, spite, selfishness, false prophecy, superstitions.	Genesis 4:5,7,8, Numbers 5:11-30, Galatians 5:19, Proverbs 10:10,12
Lying Spirit Untruthful liar, deceit.	Lies, gossips, slander, false prophesy. strong delusions, exaggeration, alse accusations, flattery, superstitions, profanity, hypocrisy, insinuation.	2 Chronicles 18:22, 2 Peter, Jeremiah 23:15,17; 1 Tim 4:7
Spirit of Heaviness Grief, anxiety, mourning	Excessive mourning, self-pity, suicidal, despair, dejection, hopelessness, broken-hearted, works with sprit of infirmity.	Isaiah 6:13, Isaiah 61:3, Luke 4:18, Psalm 69:20, Nehemiah 2:2, Mark 9

Appendix

Strongman	Fruit	Scripture Support
Perverse Spirit Distort, twist, pervert, corrupted.	Filthy mind, incest, evil actions, child abuse, pornography, twisting the Word, lust, pervert Gospel, self lovers, sexual perversion, homosexual, prostitution, false teacher, rebellion, false gender orientation.	Proverbs 2:12-15, Proverbs 23:33, Proverbs 17:20,23; Romans 1:17-32, Romans 1:30, Acts 13:10
Spirit of Pride Haughty spirit, arrogant spirit.	Pride, stubbornness, obstinate, contentious, self deception, smug, scornful	Proverbs 6:16-19, I Sam 15:23,Luke 18:11-12, Proverbs 20:1, Jeremiah 43:2
Spirit of Fear Cowardice and timidity, to be fearful causing flight	Fear of man, untrusting, stress, anxiety, torment, phobias, faithless, trembling, greed, faithless, worry, inferiority, rejection	Revelation 21:8, Isaiah 13:7-8, 1 Peter 5:7, Proverbs 29:25
Spirit of Whoredom Adultery, unfaithfulness, whoredom	Spirit, soul or body prostitution, love of money, fornication, idolatry, love of world, love of food, love of position and power, links with perverse spirits.	Ezekiel 16:15,28; Pro 5:1-14, Proverbs 15:27, Hos 4:13-19, James 4:4
Spirit of Infirmity Weakness of our human nature, sickness.	Lingering disorders, oppression, weakness, impotence, lame, bent, asthma, allergies, attention seeking, needy, frail, viruses, colds.	Luke 13:11, John 5:5, Acts 10:38, Acts 3:2, Acts 4:9
Deaf and Dumb Spirit Inability to speak, unable to hear.	Dumbness, blindness, deafness, seizures, wallowing, crying, epilepsy, hearing (natural and spiritual), ear problems.	Mark 9:17, Mark 9:22, Mark 9:18, 26; Matt 17:15, Matthew 12:22
Spirit of Bondage Slavery	Fears, addictions, bondage to sin, compulsive sin, fear of death, servant of corruption, captivity to Satan, bitterness, crushed, broken, anguish.	Romans 8:15, Romans 6:16, Hebrews 2:14-15, Acts 8:23, 2 Peter 2:19,26

Strongman	Fruit	Scripture Support
Seducing Spirit To cause to wander, lead astray, deceiving, seducing	Hypocritical lies, fascination with false prophets, wander from Truth, false signs and wonders, drawn to evil things, ways, and people, religions.	1 John 4:3, I John 1:7, 1 John 2:18-19, 22
Spirit of Anti-Christ Opposing our Christ, one who assumes a disguise of Christ, against Christ.	Denies atonement, teaches heresies, deceiver, worldly speech and actions, against our Christ and His teachings, utters blasphemies, attacks testimonies, claims authority.	John 4:3, 1 John 1:7, 1 John 2:18-19,22
Spirit of Error Wanderer, lost	Forsaking the right path, contentious, unteachable, servant of corruption, defensive, argumentative.	Proverbs 14:22, 2 Peter 2, James 3:16, Proverbs 29:1, Proverbs10:17, 2 Timothy 4:1-4, John 4:4-6
Spirit of Jezebel literally means "without cohabitation." This spirit is without gender.	Desire to control and dominate, sexual perversity, fiercely independent, and intensely ambitious, unbridled witchcraft and hatred for male authority and the prophets of God. False teacher.	Revelation 2:20, I Kings 18:4-13, I Kings 18:4-13, 1 Kings 19:1-2, Matt 14:8, Mark 6:17-18, Matt 14:3-12, I Kings 21:1-15
Spirit of Haughtiness Exaltedness	Aloof, proud, scornful, egotistic, self-righteous, controlling, bragging, gossip, contention, mockery.	Proverbs 16:18,19; Proverbs 1:22, 1 Samuel 15:23; 2 Samuel 22:8

Jesus has given us power and dominion over all these strongholds. To bind them from operating, pray for the Holy Spirit to come into the situation to set the captive free, to remove the chains that have bound and shackled, and to proclaim freedom from them in the holy and powerful name of Jesus! (Systematic Theology Outline, 1990)

Appendix B

Flat Earth Scripture References

<u>Earth created before the Sun:</u> Genesis 1:1-9

<u>Universe is complete:</u> Genesis 2:1

<u>Earth measurements unknown:</u> Job 38:4-5, Jeremiah 31:37, Proverbs 25:3

<u>Earth is a Disk/Circle, not a Ball:</u> Isaiah 40:22, Job 38:13-14

<u>Earth measured with a line, not a curve:</u> Job 38:4-5

<u>Paths are straight, not curved:</u> 1 Samuel 6:12, Psalm 5:8, Psalm 27:11, Isaiah 40:3, Jeremiah 31:9, Matthew 3:3, Mark 1:3, Luke 3:4, John 1:23, Acts 16:11, Acts 21:1, Hebrews 12:13

<u>Waters are Straight, not curved:</u> Job 37:10

<u>Earthquakes shake Earth, and does not move:</u> 2 Samuel 22:8 [This a song by David], Isaiah 13:13, Revelation 6:12-13

<u>Earth is fixed and immovable:</u> 1 Chronicles 16:30, Psalm 33:9, Psalm 93:1, Psalm 96:10, Psalm 104:5, Psalm 119:89-90, Isaiah 14:7, Isaiah 45:18, Zechariah 1:11, Luke 8:17, Hebrews 11:10, 2 Peter 3:5 [earth standing]

<u>Earth has Pillars, and hangs on nothing:</u> 1 Samuel 2:8, Job 9:6, Job 26:7, Psalm 75:3, Acts 7:49

<u>Earth has a Face (a geometrical flat surface):</u> Genesis 1:29, Genesis 4:14, Genesis 6:1, Genesis 6:7, Genesis 7:3, Genesis 7:4, Genesis 8:9, Genesis 11:8, Genesis 11:9, Genesis 41:56, Exodus 32:12, Exodus 33:16, Numbers 12:3, Deuteronomy 6:15, Deuteronomy 7:6, 1 Samuel 20:15, 1 Kings 13:34, Job 37:12, Psalm 104:30, Jeremiah 25:26, Jeremiah 28:16, Ezekiel 34:6, Ezekiel 38:20, Ezekiel 39:14, Amos 9:6, Amos 9:8, Zechariah 5:3, Luke 12:56, Luke 21:35

Waters have a Face (a geometrical flat surface): Genesis 1:2, Genesis 7:18, Job 38:30

Sky has a Face (a geometrical flat surface): Matthew 16:3, Luke 12:56

Earth has Ends: Deuteronomy 28:49, Deuteronomy 28:64, Deuteronomy 33:17, 1 Samuel 2:10, Job 37:3, Job 38:13, Psalm 46:9, Psalm 48:10, Psalm 59:13, Psalm 61:2, Psalm 65:5, Psalm 67:7, Psalm 72:8, Psalm 98:3, Psalm 135:7, Proverbs 17:24, Proverbs 30:4, Isaiah 5:26, Isaiah 26:15, Isaiah 40:28, Isaiah 41:5, Isaiah 41:9, Isaiah 42:10, Isaiah 43:6, Isaiah 45:22, Isaiah 48:20, Isaiah 49:6, Isaiah 52:10, Jeremiah 10:13, Jeremiah 16:19, Jeremiah 25:31, Jeremiah 25:33, Jeremiah 51:16, Daniel 4:22, Micah 5:4, Zechariah 9:10, Matthew 12:42, Luke 11:31, Acts 13:47

Earth has 4 Corners/Quarters: Jeremiah 9:26, Jeremiah 25:23, Isaiah 11:12, Ezekiel 7:2, Ecclesiastes 1:6, Revelation 7:1, Revelation 20:8

Earth has Foundations: Job 38:4, Psalm 82:5, Psalm 102:25 , Psalm 104:5, Proverbs 8:29, Isaiah 22:18, Isaiah 24:18, Isaiah 40:21, Isaiah 48:13, Isaiah 51:13, Isaiah 51:16, , Micah 6:2, Zechariah 12:1, Hebrews 1:10

Sun Moves, not the Earth: Genesis 15:12, Genesis 15:17, Genesis 19:23, Genesis 32:31, Exodus 17:12, Exodus 22:3, Exodus 22:26, Leviticus 22:7, Numbers 2:3, Numbers 21:11, Numbers 34:15, Deuteronomy 4:41, Deuteronomy 4:47, Deuteronomy 11:30, Deuteronomy 16:6, Deuteronomy 23:11, Deuteronomy 24:13, Deuteronomy 24:15, Joshua 1:15, Joshua 8:29, Joshua 10:27, Joshua 12:1, Joshua 13:5, Joshua 19:12, Joshua 19:27, Joshua 19:34, Judges 8:13, Judges 9:33, Judges 14:18, Judges 19:14, Judges 20:43, 2 Samuel 2:24, 2 Samuel 3:35, 2 Samuel 23:4, 1 Kings 22:36, 2 Chronicles 18:34, Psalm 50:1, Psalm 113:3, Ecclesiastes 1:5, Isaiah 41:25, Isaiah 45:6, Isaiah 59:19, Jeremiah 15:9, Daniel 6:14, Amos 8:9, Jonah 4:8, Micah 3:6, Nahum 3:17, Malachi 1:11, Matthew 5:45, Mark 16:2, Ephesians 4:26, James 1:11

Moon has its own Light: Genesis 1:16, Isaiah 13:10, Isaiah 30:26, Isaiah 60:19-20, Jeremiah 31:35, Ezekiel 32:7, Matthew 24:29, Mark 13:24, Revelation 21:23

Flat Earth Prophecy: Isaiah 40:4-5 correlates with Revelation 1:7

The (1) Firmament/Dome/Vaulted Dome, and expanse created thereby and upon where God's throne exists: Genesis 1:6-8, Genesis 1:14-18, Genesis 1:20, Genesis 7:11, Genesis 8:2, Job 9:8, Job 26:7, Job 28:24, Job 37:3, Job 37:18, Psalm 19:1, Psalm 148:4, Psalm 150:1, Proverbs 8:28, Isaiah 40:22, Isaiah 42:5, Isaiah 44:24, Isaiah 45:12, Isaiah 48:13, Ezekiel 1:22-26, Ezekiel 10:1, Daniel 12:3, Amos 9:6, Acts 7:56, Revelation 4:6, Revelation 6:14

Heliocentric Sun-god worshippers: Deuteronomy 4:19, Deuteronomy 17:3, 2 Kings 23:5, Jeremiah 8:2, Acts 7:42-43, Acts 14:8-20

Everyone Sees Yahushua: Revelation 1:7

"Breadth", spread out FLAT, of the Earth: Genesis 13:17, Job 38:18, Isaiah 8:8, Isaiah 42:5 ("spread out the earth"), Revelation 20:9

Lucifer/Satan's Conspiracy to unite the world against Yahushua's throne which is above the Firmament: Genesis 11:1-9; Psalm 2; Isaiah 14:12-15; Revelation 12:7-9

God's Word is ALWAYS Faithful and True: Jeremiah 42:5, Revelation 3:14, Revelation 19:11, Revelation 21:5, Revelation 22:6

REFERENCES

Biblegateway.com (1995 – 2017). Zondervan Corp.

BibleHub.com (2004-2023).

Brand, Paul and Yancey, Philip. (1980). *In the Likeness of God*. Grand Rapids, Michigan: Zondervan Publishing House.

Brand, Paul & Yancey, Philip. (1984). *In His Image*. Grand Rapids, Michigan: Zondervan Publishing House.

Bridges, Jerry. (2007). *Respectable Sins*. Carol Stream, Illinois: Tyndale House Publishers.

Comfort, Ray. (2001). *Scientific Facts in the Bible*. Newberry, Florida: Bridge Logos Publishers.

Frankl, Viktor E. (1959). *Man's Search for Meaning*. Boston, Massachusetts: Beacon Press.

Guillen, Michael. (2015). *Amazing Truths: How Science and the Bible Agree*. Grand Rapids, Michigan: Zondervan.

Guthrie, Nancy. (2018). *Even Better Than Eden*. Wheaton, Illinois: Crossway Publications.

Hammond, Frank & Hammond, Ida Mae. (1973). *Pigs in the Parlor*. Kirkwood, Missouri: Impact Christian Books, Inc.

Ingram, Cass. (2016). *The Cure Is in the Cupboard*. Vernon Hills, Illinois: Knowledge House Publishers.

Kelly, Matthew. (2018). *The Biggest Lie in the History of Christianity*. North Palm Beach, Florida: Eucalyptus Media Group.

Krueger, Kimberly & Nelson, Luanne. (2017). *The Miracle Effect*. Muskego, Wisconsin: FEW International Publications.

Lewis, C. S. (2016). *The Screwtape Letters*. Las Vegas, Nevada: FAB

Milam, Don. (2003). *The Ancient Language of Eden*. Shippensburg, Pennsylvania: Destiny Image Publishers, Inc.

MLS, Inc. (1990). *Systematic Theology Outline*. Sterling, Alaska: MLS Publishing.

Morris, Henry M. (1974). *Scientific Creationism*. Green Forest, Arkansas: Master Books

NAS Exhaustive Concordance of the Bible with Hebrew-Aramaic and Greek Dictionaries. Copyright © 1981, 1998 by The Lockman Foundation

Nelson, Luanne. (2020). *Daring to Believe*. Milwaukee, Wisconsin: Nico 11 Publishing and Design.

Orwell, George. (1949). *1984*. New York City, New York: Penguin Random House.

Saad, Gad. (2020). *The Parasitic Mind*. Washington, DC: Regnery Publishing.

Sanger, Laura. (2020). *The Roots of the Federal Reserve: Tracing the Nephilim from Noah to the US Dollar*. Dallas, Texas: Relentlessly Creative Books LLC.

Sproul, R.C. (2010) *Now That's a Good Question!* Carol Stream, Illinois: Tyndale Publishers, Inc.

Strobel, Lee. (2004). *The Case for a Creator*. Grand Rapids. Michigan: Zondervan.

Systematic Theology Outline. (1990). Sterling, Alaska: MLS Publishing.

All Scripture verses are from https://www.biblegateway.com using the *New American Standard Bible* unless otherwise stated.

Online References— Part One

References are in order of first occurrence.

https://biblehub.com/greek/5331.htm

Staff Writers. *Why Did God Create Us?* Got Questions Ministries. Retrieved June 10, 2022. https://www.gotquestions.org/why-did-God-create-us.html

Cartwright, Rhianna. *Why Robots Will Never Be Human: Insights into Life.* © 2022 Church of God, a Worldwide Association, Inc. Retrieved June 11, 2022. https://lifehopeandtruth.com/life/blog/why-robots-will-never-be-human/

Boyd, Greg. *Rethink Everything You Knew: Where Is Human Free Will in the Bible?* Retrieved December 13, 2018. https://reknew.org/2018/12/where-is-human-free-will-in-the-bible/

Staff Writers. *Did God Create Evil?* Got Questions Ministries. Retrieved June 10, 2022. https://www.gotquestions.org/did-God-create-evil.html/

Staff Writers, *The Spirit, Soul, and Body.* © 2019 Early Christian Beliefs. Retrieved June 10, 2022. https://earlychristianbeliefs.org/the-spirit-soul-body/

Jones, Erik. *God Places Man in the Garden of Eden.* © 2022 Church of God, a Worldwide Association, Inc. Retrieved June 12, 2022. https://lifehopeandtruth.com/bible/blog/god-places-man-in-the-garden-of-eden/

Manion, Jeff. *Beyond the Weekend: The Garden.* © 2022 Ada Bible Church. Retrieved June 10, 2022. https://www.beyondtheweekend.org/2021/11/30/november-30-the-garden/

Andres, Michael. *Between Two Gardens.* A project of the Andreas Center and Dordt University. Retrieved May 2, 2022. https://inallthings.org/between-two-gardens/

Yuan, Christopher. *He Made Them Male and Female*. Moody Bible Institute. Retrieved April 12, 2022. https://www.desiringgod.org/articles/he-made-them-male-and-female

Deyoung, Kevin. *What Does the Bible Say About Transgenderism?* TGC, The Gospel Coalition. Retrieved April 12, 2022. https://www.thegospelcoalition.org/blogs/kevin-deyoung/what-does-the-bible-say-about-transgenderism/

Margolis, Matt. *Science Says There Are Only Two Genders, No Gender 'Spectrum'.* PJ Media Poll. Retrieved April 12, 2022. https://pjmedia.com/culture/matt-margolis/2020/02/15/science-says-there-are-only-two-genders-no-gender-spectrum-n379108

https://www.kjvbible.org/firmament.html

Fass, Oren. *My Encounter with the Firmament*. Project TABS. Retrieved June 19, 2022. https://www.thetorah.com/article/my-encounter-with-the-firmament

Farber, Zev. *If the Sun Is Created on Day 4, What Is the Light on Day 1?* Project TABS. Retrieved June 19, 2022. https://www.thetorah.com/article/if-the-sun-is-created-on-day-4-what-is-the-light-on-day-1

Team Member. *Eve and the Forbidden Fruit*. Alimentarium, a Nestle Foundation. Retrieved May 10, 2022. https://www.alimentarium.org/en/fact-sheet/eve-and-forbidden-fruit

Hempel, Charlotte. *The Society for Old Testament Study*. Retrieved May 10, 2022. https://www.sots.ac.uk/

Calahan, John. *Never Thirsty*. Like the Master Ministries. Retrieved May 17, 2022. https://www.neverthirsty.org/bible-qa/qa-archives/question/was-the-serpent-the-only-animal-that-talked-in-the-garden-of-eden/

Bouchard, Karen Scalf. *7 Interesting Things You May Not Have Considered About the Garden of Eden*. Biblica. Retrieved, May 30,

2022. https://www.biblica.com/articles/7-interesting-things-you-may-not-have-considered-about-the-garden-of-eden/

Staff Writer. *How much time passed in the Bible between the time of Adam and Eve and the time of Noah?* Retrieved May 30, 2022. https://www.quora.com/How-much-time-passed-in-the-Bible-between-the-time-of-Adam-and-Eve-and-the-time-of-Noah

Biblegateway. *Lockyer's All the Men of the Bible - Abram, Abraham.* Retrieved May 30, 2022. https://www.biblegateway.com/resources/all-men-bible/Abram-Abraham

Guzik, David. *Genesis 3 – Man's Temptation and Fall.* David Guzik Bible Commentary. Retrieved July 25, 2022. https://enduringword.com/bible-commentary/genesis-3/

Van Roekel, Jessica. *9 Things to Know About the Fall of Man.* Crosswalk.com. Retrieved May 29, 2022. https://www.crosswalk.com/faith/bible-study/things-to-know-about-the-fall-of-man.html

Kastrup, Bernardo. *Yes, Free Will Exists.* Scientific American, a Division of Nature America Inc. Retrieved June 3, 2022. https://blogs.scientificamerican.com/observations/yes-free-will-exists/

McLeod, Saul. *Freewill vs Determinism.* Simply Scholar, Ltd. Retrieved June 1, 2022. https://www.simplypsychology.org/freewill-determinism.html

Staff Writer. *What is Spiritual Death? What does it Mean to be Spiritually Dead?* Got Questions Ministries. Retrieved May 15, 2022. https://www.compellingtruth.org/spiritually-dead.html

Bradford. Alina. *Science and the Scientific Method.* Future US, Inc. Retrieved May 10, 2022. https://www.livescience.com/20896-science-scientific-method.html

Bradford, Alina. *What is Scientific Hypothesis?* Future US, Inc. Retrieved May 10, 2022. https://www.livescience.com/20896-science-scientific-method.html

Robey, Charles (Chuck). *The Tower of Babel Revised.* Christian Living, FaithWriters.com Retrieved June 3, 2022. https://www.faithwriters.com/article-details.php?id=200587

Griffin, Annette. *The Tower of Babel – Bible Story.* Retrieved June 3, 2022. https://www.biblestudytools.com/bible-stories/the-tower-of-babel.html.

Staff Writer. *Chapter 4.* Retrieved July 25, 2022. https://www.biblestudytools.com/history/flavius-josephus/antiquities-jews/book-1/chapter-4.html

Lickerman, Alex. *Why We Need to Know Why.* Psychology Today. Retrieved June 3, 2022. https://www.psychologytoday.com/us/blog/happiness-in-world/201011/why-we-need-know-why

Bolinger, Hope. *What Sunday School Did Not Teach You About the Tree of Knowledge.* Crosswalk.com. Retrieved June 3, 2022. https://www.crosswalk.com/faith/bible-study/what-sunday-school-didnt-teach-you-about-the-tree-of-knowledge.html\

Smyth, Delores. *Why Was Lucifer, Satan, Cast Out of Heaven and Banished to Hell?* Crosswalk Ministries. Retrieved July 10, 2022. https://www.crosswalk.com/faith/bible-study/why-was-satan-banished-in-the-bible.html

Promise Keepers Manager. *What Does Satan Want?* Retrieved July 10, 2022. https://promisekeepers.org/what-does-satan-want/

Online References–Part Two
References are in order of first occurrence.

Shirley, Steve. *Can Satan (or His Demons) Create Things or Take on Human Form?* JesusAlive.cc. Retrieved July 7, 2022. https://jesusalive.cc/can-satan-create/.

Oakes, John. *If God Regretted Making Human Beings (Genesis 6:6), Does This Mean That God Made a Mistake? What Does This*

Say About God? Evidence for Christianity. Retrieved July 8, 2022. https://evidenceforchristianity.org/if-god-regretted-making-human-beings-genesis-66-does-this-mean-that-god-made-a-mistake-what-does-this-say-about-god/.

Turner, Jill Foley. *God's Generosity: A Reason to Know We Can Trust Him.* National Christian Foundation. Retrieved July 8, 2022. https://www.ncfgiving.com/stories/the-generosity-of-god/.

Staff Writers. *What Is Pharmakeia in the Bible?* Got Questions Ministries. Retrieved July 12, 2022. https://www.gotquestions.org/pharmakeia-in-the-Bible.html

Shine, Bernie. *The Art of Deception: A Magician's View.* Huffpost.com. Retrieved July 12, 2022. https://www.huffpost.com/entry/the-art-of-deception-a-ma_b_8161274.

https://www.merriam-webster.com/dictionary/sorcery

Staff Writer, *Job and Work, Introduction to Job.* Bible Commentary Produced by the TOW Project. https://www.theologyofwork.org/old-testament/job/jobs-friends-blame-job-for-the-calamity-job-4-23/jobs-friends-accuse-him-of-doing-evil-job-4-23

Bird, Chad. *Three Hidden Hebrew Treasures in Psalm 23.* 1517. Christ for You. Retrieved July 20, 2022. https://www.1517.org/articles/three-hidden-hebrew-treasures-in-psalm-23

Piper, Barnabas. *4 Things the Old Testament Teaches About Suffering.* Crosswalk.com. Retrieved July 20, 2022. https://www.crosswalk.com/faith/bible-study/4-things-the-old-testament-teaches-about-suffering.html

Zavada, Jack. *Introduction to the Book of Zechariah: The Messiah Is Coming.* LearnReligions.com. Retrieved July 20, 2022. https://www.learnreligions.com/book-of-zechariah-4036303

Conley, John. *The Truth About Magic, Witchcraft and Sorcery.* BelieversWeb.org. Retrieved July 12, 2022. https://believersweb.org/the-truth-about-magic-witchcraft-and-sorcery/

Ritenbaugh, John W. *What Sin Is and What Sin Does*. Church of the Great God. Retrieved July 20, 2022. https://www.cgg.org/index. cfm/library/article/id/489/what-sin-is-does.htm

Armstrong, Herbert. *Were the Ten Commandments in Force Before Moses?* Church of the Great God. Retrieved July 20, 2022. https:// www.cgg.org/index.cfm/library/booklet/id/744/were-ten-commandments-before-moses.htm.

Lockwood, Burt. *The Timeline Between Adam and Jesus*. Blogos. org. Blogging God's Word. Retrieved July 20, 2022. https://www. blogos.org/exploringtheword/adam-Jesus-timeline.php.

Staff Writer. *Biblical Prophesies Fulfilled by Jesus*. CBN. Christian Broadcasting Network. Retrieved July 26, 2022. https://www1.cbn. com/biblestudy/biblical-prophecies-fulfilled-by-jesus.

Schrock, David. *Darkness: The World in Which Christ was Born*. David Schrock Ministries. Retrieved July 26, 2022. https:// davidschrock.com/2011/12/12/darkness-the-world-in-which-christ-was-born/

Staff Writer. *What Changes Happened After Pentecost?* Ligonier Ministries. Retrieved July 25, 2022. https://www.christianity.com/ jesus/early-church-history/pentecost/what-changes-happened-after-penecost.html

Guzik, David. *Acts 19 – Paul in Ephesus*. David Guzik Bible Commentary. Retrieved July 25, 2022. https://enduringword.com/ bible-commentary/acts-19/

Martin, Ernest. *Simon Magus (Simon THE PATER) Founder of the Roman Catholic Church*. http://www.pointsoftruth.com/ SimonMagus.html reposted on LiveJournal.com. Retrieved June 1, 2022. https://archangel16.livejournal.com/180135.html

Lujack, George. *Catholicism's First Pope: Simon Magus*. Scripture Truth Ministries. Retrieved June 1, 2022. http:// scripturetruthministries.com/2018/03/26/catholicisms-first-pope-simon-magus/

Guzik, David. *Matthew 16 – Revealing Who Jesus Is and What He Came To Do.* David Guzik Bible Commentary. Retrieved July 25, 2022. https://enduringword.com/bible-commentary/matthew-16/

Haynes, Clarence L., Jr. *8 Facts About Satan You Need to Know.* Crosswalk.com. Retrieved July 23, 2022. https://www.crosswalk.com/faith/bible-study/facts-about-satan-you-need-to-know.html

Staff Writer. *Satan is god.* Unknown. Retrieved July, 25, 2022. https://satanisgod.org/

Sausedo, Alejandro. *Most Don't Know This About Satan.* 3n1 Ministry. Retrieved July 15, 2022. https://www.facebook.com/watch/?v=722475555567045

Guzik, David. *Mark 1 – The Beginning of the Gospel.* David Guzik Bible Commentary. Retrieved July 25, 2022. https://enduringword.com/bible-commentary/mark-1/

Staff Writer. *Who Can Cast Out Demons?* Deliverance Ministry Network. Retrieved July 15, 2022. http://www.ministeringdeliverance.com/who_cast_demons.php

Cole, Graham A. *10 Things You Should Know About Demons and Satan.* Crossway Ministries. Retrieved July 12, 2022. https://www.crossway.org/articles/10-things-you-should-know-about-demons/

Muther, Christopher. *Welcome to Tel Aviv, the Gayest City on Earth.* Retrieved July 20, 2022. https://www.bostonglobe.com/lifestyle/travel/2016/03/17/welcome-tel-aviv-gayest-city-earth/y9V15VazXhtSjXVSo9gT9K/story.html

Guzik, David. *Genesis 27 – Jacob Deceptively Gains the Blessing of Isaac.* David Guzik Bible Commentary. Retrieved July 25, 2022. https://enduringword.com/bible-commentary/genesis-27/

Staff Writer. *History of the Khazarians, Today's Jews.* Jew World Order. Retrieved January 5, 2022. https://www.jewworldorder.org/history-khazarians-todays-jews/

Harris, Mike. *Hidden History of the Incredibly Evil Khazarian Mafia.* Covert Geopolitics. Retrieved January 5, 2022. https://geopolitics.co/2015/03/11/hidden-history-of-the-incredibly-evil-khazarian-mafia/

James, Preston. *The Hidden History of the Incredibly Evil Khazarian Mafia.* Veterans Today. Retrieved January 5, 2022. https://www.veteranstoday.com/2022/03/10/the-hidden-history-of-the-incredibly-evil-khazarian-mafia/

https://amazon.com/Thirteenth-Tribe-Khazar

Staff Writer. *Bit of Khazarian History in Relation to the Takeover of Russia by the Khazarians in 1917 With Continuing Ramifications Today.* Jew World Order. Retrieved January 5, 2022. https://www.jewworldorder.org/bit-of-khazarian-history-in-relation-to-the-takeover-of-russia-by-the-khazarians-in-1917-with-continuing-ramifications-today/

Watkins, Donald V. The Rothschilds: Controlling the World's Money Supply for More Than Two Centuries. Retrieved 2,2022. https://www.donaldwatkins.com/post/the-rothschilds-controlling-the-world-s-money-supply-for-more-than-two-centuries

Carleton, John. *Bit of Khazarian History in Relation to the Takeover of Russia by the Khazarians in 1917 With Continuing Ramifications Today*. Retrieved January 3, 2022. https://www.johnccarleton.org/BLOGGER/2022/02/27/bit-of-khazarian-history-in-relation-to-the-takeover-of-russia-by-the-khazarians-in-1917/

Marrs, Tex. *DNA Research Confirms That Modern Khazarian "Jews" Are Not the Descendants of Ancient Isrealites or The Seed of Abraham.* Retrieved January 3, 2022. https://educate-yourself.org/cn/texemarrskhazarianjews08mar13.shtml

Preston, James and Harris, Mike. *Hidden History of the Incredibly Evil Khazarian Mafia.* Retrieved January 4, 2022. https://

geopolitics.co/2015/03/11/hidden-history-of-the-incredibly-evil-khazarian-mafia/

Online References—Part Three

References are in order of first occurrence.

https://abbreviations.yourdictionary.com/articles/what-do-bc-and-ad-stand-for-dates-in-history.html

Hunter, Todd. *Our Top 5 Temptations*. Faith Gateway. Retrieved July 17, 2022. https://faithgateway.com/blogs/christian-books/our-top-five-temptations/

Staff Writer. *Genetically Modified Foods*. World Health Organization (WHO). Retrieved July 15, 2022. https://www.who.int/news-room/questions-and-answers/item/food-genetically-modified

Smith, Jeffrey. *Will Genetically Modified Foods Make You Sick?* Institute for Responsible Technology. Retrieved July 22, 2022. (https://www.huffpost.com/entry/will-genetically-modified_b_145320)

Barrett, Mike. *Worldwide GMO Labeling Laws*. Occupy.com Retrieved July 20, 2022. https://www.occupy.com/article/worldwide-gmo-labeling-laws

Staff Writer. *World Rivers Polluted With Drugs*. Tomorrow's World. Retrieved July 17, 2022. https://www.tomorrowsworld.org/news-and-prophecy/world-rivers-polluted-with-drugs

Staff Writer. *What Are They Spraying in the Sky?* The City Edition. Retrieved July 17, 2022. https://chemtrailsafety.com/chemtrails_contrails.html

Missler, Chuck. *The Federal Reserve System: It's Not "Federal" and There's No "Reserve"*. The Millennium Report. Retrieved July 20,

2022. https://themillenniumreport.com/2017/12/the-federal-reserve-system-its-not-federal-and-theres-no-reserve/

Staff Writer. *Who Controls the Money Controls the World.* We Hold These Truths (WHTT). Retrieved July 20, 2022. https://whtt.org/who-controls-the-money-controls-the-world/

https://www.thewealthrecord.com/about/

Evans, Tony. *Do You Believe God's Word?* Tony Evans The Urban Alternative. Retrieved July 20, 2022. https://tonyevans.org/blog/do-you-believe-gods-word

Deyoung, Kevin. *3 Things we Must Believe About God's Word.* TGC, The Gospel Coalition. Retrieved July 22, 2022. https://www.crossway.org/articles/3-things-we-must-believe-about-gods-word/

Steven, J. *15 NASA Research Papers That Admit Flat & Nonrotating!* The Bible Bet. Retrieved January 20, 2022. https://www.galileolied.com/post/15-nasa-research-papers-admit-flat-nonrotating

Staff Writer, *A Mathematical Model of the Ch-53 Helicopter.* NASA.gov. Retrieved January 20, 2022. https://ntrs.nasa.gov/citations/19810003557

Peer-to-Peer Content Sharing Platform. *NASA = SATAN.* Platobel, Odysee.com. Retrieved January 20, 2022. https://www.bitchute.com/video/dGsFNuetkP5o/

Pritchard, Tommy. *NASA's Dark Origins.* Futurism.com. Retrieved January 20, 2022. https://vocal.media/futurism/nasa-s-dark-origins

Klein, Christopher. *10 Things You May Not Know About John D. Rockefeller.* History.com. Retrieved July 25, 2022. https://www.history.com/news/10-things-you-may-not-know-about-john-d-rockefeller

Allison E., Mandler B. *Non-fuel Products of Oil and Gas.* American Geosciences Institute. Retrieved July 25, 2022. https://www.americangeosciences.org/geoscience-currents/non-fuel-products-oil-and-gas

References

Editors of Encyclopedia Britannica, updated by Amy Tikkanen. *IG Farben.* Britannica.com. Retrieved July 25, 2022. https://www.britannica.com/topic/IG-Farben

Sharav, Vera Hassner. *Auschwitz: 60 Year Anniversary– the Role of IG Farben-Bayer.* ALLIANCE FOR HUMAN RESEARCH PROTECTION, Advancing Voluntary, Informed Consent to Medical Intervention. Retrieved, July 25, 2022. https://ahrp.org/auschwitz60-year-anniversary-the-role-of-ig-farben-bayer/

Schmidt, Eric. *How Rockefeller Created the Business of Western Medicine.* Meridian Health Clinic. Retrieved July 25, 2022. https://meridianhealthclinic.com/how-rockefeller-created-the-business-of-western-medicine/

Freeman, Makia. *How John D. Rockefeller Used the AMA to Take Over Western Medicine.* The Liberty Beacon. Retrieved July 25, 2022. https://www.thelibertybeacon.com/john-d-rockefeller-used-ama-take-western-medicine/

Gustav, Kuhn. *Tricking the Brain: How Magic Works.* TheConversation.com. Retrieved June 10, 2022. https://theconversation.com/tricking-the-brain-how-magic-works-56451

Staff Writer. *Cognitive Dissonance.* Psychology Today. Retrieved July 20, 2022. https://www.psychologytoday.com/us/basics/cognitive-dissonance

Staff Writer. *Medical Protocol Definition.* LawInsider.com Retrieved July 25, 2022. https://www.lawinsider.com/dictionary/medical-protocol

Staff Writer. *American Academy of Pediatrics' New Guidelines Support Gender Change for Kids.* LifeSiteNews.com Retrieved August 3, 2022. https://www.lifesitenews.com/news/american-academy-of-pediatrics-new-guidelines-support-gender-change-for-kid/

Madara, James L. *AMA to States: Stop Interfering in Health Care of Transgender Children.* American Medical Association (AMA).

Retrieved August 6, 2022. https://www.ama-assn.org/press-center/press-releases/ama-states-stop-interfering-health-care-transgender-children

Staff Writer. *Gender Affirmation (Confirmation) or Sex Reassignment Surgery.* ClevelandClinic.org. Retrieved June 6, 2022. https://my.clevelandclinic.org/health/treatments/21526-gender-affirmation-confirmation-or-sex-reassignment-surgery

Fontanilla. Kali. *Teachers Who Don't Affirm Gender Identities Accused of Harming Students.* The EpochTimes.com. Retrieved August 27, 2022. https://www.theepochtimes.com/teachers-who-dont-affirm-gender-identities-accused-of-harming-students_4691405.html

Saad, Lydia. *How Many Americans Believe in God?* Gallup.com. Retrieved July 15, 2022. https://news.gallup.com/poll/268205/americans-believe-god.aspx

Kearney, Melissa. *The Mystery of the Declining Birth Rate.* The Econofact Network. Retrieved July 30, 2022. https://econofact.org/the-mystery-of-the-declining-u-s-birth-rate

Ray, Siladitya. *Abortion Rates in the U.S. Rose in 2020 After 30 Years of Decline, Report Says.*

Forbes.com. Retrieved August 6, 2022. https://www.forbes.com/sites/siladityaray/2022/06/15/abortion-rates-in-the-us-rose-in-2020-after-30-years-of-decline-report-says/?sh=735ccd576985

Staff Writer. *Abortion Statistics.* American Life League (All.com). Retrieved August 6, 2022. https://www.all.org/abortion/abortion-statistics

Blood Ranger. *Could Artificial Intelligence be Satan?* Geeks and Gamers. Retrieved August 16, 2022. https://www.geeksandgamers.com/topic/could-artificial-intelligence-be-satan/

Waddell, Allan. *Injecting Artificial Intelligence with Empathy.* The Ethics Centre. Retrieved August 22, 2022. https://ethics.org.au/injecting-artificial-intelligence-with-human-empathy/

References

Bradshaw, Peter. *The Minority Report*. The Guardian. Retrieved August 22, 2022. https://www.theguardian.com/film/2002/jun/28/culture.reviews

Dornik, Jeff. *Artificial Intelligence is Being Injected Into Humans. Is This the Return of the Genesis 6 Nephilim?* Freedom First Network. Retrieved August 22, 2022. https://freedomfirstnetwork.com/2022/09/artificial-intelligence-is-being-injected-into-humans-is-this-the-return-of-the-genesis-6-nephilim

Hinchliffe, Tim. *Yuval Harari's Hackable Humans*. The Sociable. Retrieved August 22, 2022. *https://sociable.co/military-technology/yuval-harari-hackable-humans-wef-darpa-preconscious-brain-signals/*

Staff Writer. *NIH: The Brain Initiative*. National Institute of Health. Retrieved August 22. 2022. https://braininitiative.nih.gov/strategic-planning/brain-2025-report

Chen, Hui. *An Overview of Micronanoswarms for Biomedical Applications*. American Chemistry Society (ACS). Retrieved August 22, 2022. https://pubs.acs.org/doi/10.1021/acsnano.1c07363

Staff Writer. *COVID-19 Vaccine: SPIKEVAX (Elasomeran)*. AU Government, Dept. of Health and Aged Care. Retrieved August 25, 2022. https://www.tga.gov.au/news/news/covid-19-vaccine-spikevax-elasomeran

Stolworthy, Yvonne. *Can the mRNA Vaccines Change DNA?* Medical Daily. Retrieved August 25, 2022. https://www.medicaldaily.com/can-mra-vaccine-change-dna-459011

Moore, Art. *'Health Nightmare': Dr. Robert Malone Spotlights Study on mRNA Spike Protein*. WND News Center. https://www.wndnewscenter.org/health-nightmare-dr-robert-malone-spotlights-study-on-mrna-spike-protein/

Staff Writer. *Dr David Martin*. The Totality of Evidence. Retrieved August 22, 2022. https://totalityofevidence.com/dr-david-martin/

Mercola, Joseph. *Patents Prove SARS-CoV-2 Is a Manufactured Virus.* Citizens Journal.US. Retrieved August 30, 2022. https://www. citizensjournal.us/patents-prove-sars-cov-2-is-a-manufactured-virus/

Brown, Tim. *Want to See the Effects of the COVID Shots In Autopsies? This Scientist Shows You (Video).* The Citizens Journal, Ventura County. Retrieved August 22, 2022. https://www.citizensjournal. us/want-to-see-the-effects-of-the-covid-shots-in-autopsies-this-scientist-shows-you-video/

Staff Writer. *Dr. Malone: 'Highly Vaccinated' Suffering Worse Outcomes Than Those with 'Natural Immunity'.* World Tribune. com. Retrieved August 29, 2022. https://www.worldtribune.com/ dr-malone-highly-vaccinated-suffering-worse-outcomes-than-those-with-natural-immunity/

Staff Writer. *Covid Vaccines: How Fast Is Progress Around the World?* BBC News. Retrieved August 22, 2022. https://www.bbc. com/news/world-56237778

Adams, Mike. *The Vast Majority of Pharmacology, Psychiatry, Vaccine Science, and Published Research Is a Complete Fraud.* Retrieved August 2, 2022. https://www.naturalnews.com/2022-07-29-vast-majority-of-pharmacology-science-published-research-is-a-complete-fraud.html

Parker, J. Emory. *See How Much Covid-19 Relief Money Health Care Providers in Your State Got.* STAT. Retrieved August 26, 2022. https://www.statnews.com/2021/09/24/covid-19-relief-money-providers-in-your-state/

Staff Writer. *World Population to Reach 8 Billion on 15 November 2022.* United Nations, Department of Economic and Social Affairs. Retrieved August 22, 2022. https://www.un.org/en/desa/world-population-reach-8-billion-15-november-2022

Allen, Garland E. *"Culling the Herd": Eugenics and the Conservation Movement in the United States, 1900-1940.* PubMed.gov. Retrieved August 30, 2022. https://pubmed.ncbi.nlm.nih.gov/22411125/

References

https://www.facebook.com/3n1Ministry/
videos/722475555567045

Conley, John. *The Truth About Magic, Witchcraft and Sorcery.*
BelieversWeb.org. https://believersweb.org/the-truth-about-
magic-witchcraft-and-sorcery/

Staff Writer. *How Should a Christian View Prescription Drugs?*
GotQuestions.org. Retrieved April 22, 2022. https://www.
gotquestions.org/Christian-prescription-drugs.html

Starnes, Todd. *SHOCK VIDEO: Planned Parenthood Sells Dead
Baby Body Parts.* foxnews.com. Retrieved September 3, 2022.
https://www.foxnews.com/opinion/shock-video-planned-
parenthood-sells-dead-baby-body-parts

Peters, Stew. *Top Secret Pfizer Documents Leaked: Pfizer Knew That
Vaxx Would Kill Thousands.* Stew Peters Show. Redvoicemedia.
com. Retrieved September 3, 2022. https://www.redvoicemedia.
com/2022/03/top-secret-pfizer-documents-leaked-pfizer-knew-
that-vaxx-would-kill-thousands/

Eckman, Jim. *The Victorious Church of Jesus Christ: Iran and
China.* Issues in Perspective. Retrieved September 7, 2022. http://
issuesinperspective.com/2021/08/the-victorious-church-of-jesus-
christ-iran-and-china/

Staff Writer. *PHARMAKEIA AND SORCERY. SafeguardYourSoul.
com. Retrieved September 12, 2022. https://safeguardyoursoul.com/
pharmakeia-and-sorcery/*

Fulford, Benjamin. *Worldwide Arrest Warrant for David
Rockefeller Jr. as Khazarian Mafia Take Down Continues.*
TheGoodlyLawfulSociety.com. Retrieved September 15, 2022.
https://thegoodlylawfulsociety.org/worldwide-arrest-warrant-for-
david-rockefeller-jr-as-khazarian-mafia-take-down-continues-by-
benjamin-fulford/

Appendix A Reference:

Systematic Theology Outline. (1990). Sterling, Alaska: MLS Publishing.

Appendix B References:

Staff Writer. *Flat Earth.* World's Last Chance Ministries. https://www.worldslastchance.com/biblical-christian-beliefs/flat-earth-bible-verses-more-than-200.html

https://www.openbible.info/topics/flat_earth

75 Bible Verses Prove a Flat Earth (KJV) VIDEO: https://www.youtube.com/watch?v=JKQsUsgz9AY

CPSIA information can be obtained
at www.ICGtesting.com
Printed in the USA
LVHW010419150723
752289LV00039B/1542/J